PRINCIPIA

KETOGENICA

MMXIV

Meh... "

The reference manual for nutrition health researchers,
and geeky carb dodgers.

Gramercy

This project only possible due to unquestioning support and patience of E.G. during long

stints of arduous research, sabotaged circadian rhythyms, dark nights of the ethanol-fuelled

soul, and pecuniary nodus.

Without such altruism this would have taken years longer and its fate likely yet another

forgotten part-time pet project, one more "if only" footnote.

D0451157

Contents

Introduction

Some smart guy was once paraphrased as saying something about making things as simple as possible, but no simpler. This compendium is an exercise in that philosophy.

A reductionist approach to convey complex principles which are covered across thousands of papers into a cohesive and semi-casually readable format can be challenging. Indeed in some of the papers referenced, they themselves contain hundreds of references, but the line must be drawn somewhere to avert a perpetual pursuit. It is implored that the reader follow the rabbit down the hole back to the provided sources to get a thorough comprehension on any subjects they find compelling.

Many hundreds of papers are exploratory and offer theories, in here the focus is more toward tangible outcomes rather than much discussion of the possibilities, or outlining of the biochemistry.

Papers are presented chronologically in each general section, and some of the early material whilst perhaps naive compared to modern science, is included to demonstrate the colourful history of research on these topics.

The one area in which ketogenic diets have been extensively researched and written about previously is with regard to epilepsy, thus it makes an appearance as not much more than a footnote in this book, else it would likely quadruple the length of the references section. If seizure control is of specific interest it is suggested the reader seek out existing books on the topic.

The definition of carbohydrate intake levels seems at the

complete whimsy of researchers, often with no supplied context as to how one defines subjective terms such as "high" and "low". Many papers equate anything under about ~45% of total intake being carbohydrate to be "low". For this reason much of the self-reported intake nomenclature within the literature has been ignored in favour of seeking out the actual amounts administered in the methods, and instead a basic guide to carbohydrate intake levels has been applied across the board.

General guidelines applied for carbohydrate intakes:

Definition	% of calories	Absolute amount
Very Low/Ketogenic	0-9%	0-50g
Low	10-20%	50-100g
Moderate	20-40%	100-200g
Standard/Western	40-60%	200-400g
High	>60%	>400g

Often there will be some overlap between definitions, but as it stands this guideline is satisfactory.

Disclaimer

The information provided herein is as a resource for personal research. This material does not constitute medical nor diet advice - it is presented as is.

Consult a doctor and/or professional nutritionist/dietician before embarking on any significant lifestyle or diet detour.

(Doctors and dietitians unaware of the myriad possible benefits of carbohydrate restriction should definitely have this book for their own research.)

Very Low Carbohydrate and Ketogenic Diet Research Papers

11 subjects were prescribed a diet of 300-600ml of milk and as much meat, fish, eggs, cheese, butter, margarine, cream and leafy vegetables as they wished. The amount of carbohydrate in other food was limited to not more than 50g. Average energy intake was ~1,560 calories per day, a spontaneous reduction to ~67% of baseline.

Subjects did not complain of hunger, some reporting increased well-being and better energy.

One subject very well represented the mean reduced total intake to 65%, but still consumed 90% of the usual protein, and over 100% of most nutrients as a baseline diet. The exception was calcium which also reduced to 61% in line with total intake, whereas if macronutrient composition were kept static at this level of energy intake it would result in reduction to ~65% in nutrients across the board.

The low carbohydrate diet presents no health hazard, either generally or in regard to its nutritional value. The nutrient content is appreciably higher than could be achieved by a diet in which the same caloric reduction was effected by a general restriction in all foods.

Nutrient Intake of Subjects on Low Carbohydrate Diet Used in Treatment of Obesity. - 1970

In normal subjects on a formula diet with constant carbohydrate and protein intake, the fat content was raised continuously up to a daily ingestion of more than 6,800 fat calories. There was only a slight weight gain, considering the significant excess caloric intake.

Based on these results, obese subjects were treated with high fat, low carbohydrate diets. If the carbohydrate content of the diet was not more than 50 to 60g and the fat content approximately 150g, an average daily weight reduction of 0.3 kg was achieved.

The cholesterol and triglyceride concentrations in the serum, which had been raised at the beginning of the experiment, invariably showed a tendency towards normalisation under this dietary program.

Response of body weight to a low carbohydrate, high fat diet in normal and obese subjects. - 1973

A test meal containing gelatin plus glucose resulted in much higher levels of insulin and increased insulin-glucagon ratio, lower glucagon levels, and slightly higher triglycerides than a meal of the same size of gelatin alone.

One week of very low carbohydrate ~2,800 calorie diet lowered insulin, the insulin-glucagon ratio, and triglycerides, plus increased glucagon.

Swapping back ~390g of carbohydrate significantly increased insulin, the insulin-glucagon ratio, and triglycerides, and lowered glucagon within two days; even greater disturbance of hormones were observed when increased to ~510g of carbohydrate.

Basal and postprotein insulin and glucagon levels during a high and low carbohydrate intake and their relationships to plasma triglycerides. - 1975

Two very low calorie diets were studied, one high in fat and low in carbohydrate content, the other high in carbohydrate and low in fat.

The high fat-low carbohydrate diet resulted in a greater weight loss during the 2-week observation period, then significant rapid weight gain and urinary retention of sodium in subjects who returned to a maintenance diet.

Fasting triglyceride and cholesterol levels declined to a greater extent following the high fat regimen. These changes reflected decrements in VLDL alone.

Effect of diet composition on metabolic adaptations to hypocaloric nutrition: comparison of high carbohydrate and high fat isocaloric diets. - 1977

5 well-trained cyclists were fed a weight maintenance ketogenic diet.

Maximal oxygen uptake (VO2max) was unchanged from baseline after 3 weeks.

Endurance time for continuous exercise to exhaustion at 2/3 of VO2max was much the same after 4 weeks of keto, with a three-fold drop in glucose oxidation and a four-fold reduction in muscle glycogen use.

Aerobic endurance exercise by well-trained cyclists was not compromised by four weeks of ketosis.

The human metabolic response to chronic ketosis without caloric restriction: preservation of submaximal exercise capability with reduced carbohydrate oxidation. - 1983

To study the metabolic effects of ketosis without weight

loss, nine lean men were fed a balanced diet for one week followed by four weeks of a ketogenic diet.

Diets had the same calories and protein levels, the remaining calories in the balanced diet consisting of ⅔ carbohydrate and ⅓ fat, the ketogenic diet being primarily fat with less than 20g carbohydrate.

- Weight and whole-body potassium did not vary significantly during the five-week study.
- Nitrogen balance was regained after one week on keto.
- Fasting blood glucose remained slightly lower during keto, glucose oxidation rate fell significantly.
- Serum cholesterol levels rose, while triglycerides fell.
- No disturbance of liver or kidney function was noted at the end.

The human metabolic response to chronic ketosis without caloric restriction: physical and biochemical adaptation. - 1983

Subjects overate different diets for 30 days by 1,000 calories a day more than they needed to maintain weight.

On a standard American or a high carbohydrate diet they gained ~2.7kg, however on a high fat diet they only gained ~1.75kg.

Adaptation to overeating in lean and overweight men and women. - 1983

During 14-day experimental periods, distance runners were put on a diet of either high carb or high fat.

On the high carb diet HDL cholesterol decreased, total and LDL cholesterol initially decreased but subsequently exceeded pre-diet values, while triglycerides increased significantly.

The high fat diet had little effect on total and LDL cholesterol, whereas triglycerides decreased. It provided ~111g of saturated fat per day.

The effects of high-carbohydrate and high-fat diets on the serum lipid and lipoprotein concentrations of endurance athletes. - 1984

6 healthy females in a free-living condition were put on a ketogenic diet.

Functional residual capacity (lung volume) was increased, respiratory gas exchange ratio fell (indicating increased fat oxidation), and there was a reduction in carbon dioxide production and arterial carbon dioxide tension.

An analysis of ambulatory electroencephalogram showed that REM latency increased with no significant changes in sleep time and stages.

A low carbohydrate isoenergetic diet is perfectly tolerable, influences sleep behavior, reduces carbon dioxide production and respiratory gas exchange ratio, and may be therapeutically useful in patients with hypercapnic respiratory failure.

Effects of a low carbohydrate isoenergetic diet on sleep behavior and pulmonary functions in healthy female adult humans. - 1986

7 patients with elevated cholesterol followed a diet in which most of the calories came from beef fat.

Their diets contained no sucrose, milk, or grains. They were given nutritional supplements.

Triglyceride levels decreased from ~113 to ~74, cholesterol levels fell from ~263 to ~189.

6 of the patients started with a HDL percentage of ~21%, which rose to ~32%.

Reducing the serum cholesterol level with a diet high in animal fat. - 1988

5 subjects participated in randomized crossover studies of either fasting or a lipid emulsion infusion to meet energy requirements for 84 hours.

Changes in plasma glucose, free fatty acids, ketone bodies, insulin, and epinephrine concentrations were the same in both the fasting and fed studies. These results demonstrate that restriction of dietary carbohydrate, not the general absence of energy intake itself, is responsible for the some of the benefits of short-term fasting.

Carbohydrate restriction regulates the adaptive response to fasting. - 1992

The effects of 2 weeks of either a high-fat or a high-carbohydrate diet on exercise performance in trained cyclists shows time to exhaustion during high intensity exercise was not significantly different between trials, nor were the rates of muscle glycogen utilization.

Despite a lower muscle glycogen content at the onset of moderate intensity exercise, time to exhaustion was significantly longer after the high fat diet.

Enhanced endurance in trained cyclists during moderate intensity exercise

8 healthy untrained men aged ~22 spent 3 days on a control, mixed, or a ketogenic diet of equal energy content.

In comparison with the normal diet, the ketogenic diet resulted in an increased VO2 max, decreased respiratory exchange ratio, and a shift of lactate threshold towards higher exercise loads.

On keto the blood lactate concentrations were lower before, during and after exercise. Post exercise blood pH, as well as pre-and post exercise base excess and bicarbonates were reduced. Resting ketone body concentration was elevated, during a 1h recovery period ketones decreased, while plasma free fatty acids did not change.

Both the pre-and post-exercise levels of adrenaline, noradrenaline, and cortisol were enhanced, whilst insulin concentration was decreased on the ketogenic diet.

Effect of low-carbohydrate-ketogenic diet on metabolic and hormonal responses to graded exercise in men. - 1996

6 adolescents, aged 12 to 15 years, weighing an average of ~148kg with an average BMI of ~51, were put on an energy restricted diet of ~700 calories, 25g of each fat and carbs, the rest of which derived from protein. A ketogenic regime commonly known as a protein sparing modified fast.

After 8 weeks the subjects lost ~15kg, predominantly

fat. Lean body mass was not significantly affected. Blood chemistries remained normal and included a decrease in cholesterol. Sleep abnormalities were reduced, with an increase in rapid eye movement sleep and a decrease in slow-wave sleep.

The effects of a high-protein, low-fat, ketogenic diet on adolescents with morbid obesity: body composition, blood chemistries, and sleep abnormalities. - 1998

51 children with epilepsy were put on a ketogenic diet, after 3 months about half had their frequency of seizures decreased by over 50%.

A multicenter study of the efficacy of the ketogenic diet. - 1998

16 endurance-trained cyclists were assigned to consume either their habitual diet or a high fat diet.

Consuming the high fat diet for as little as 5 to 10 days significantly alters substrate utilization (burn more fat, less sugar) during submaximal (endurance) exercise, but does not reduce performance in high intensity exercise.

Metabolic adaptations to a high-fat diet in endurance cyclists - 1999

24 subjects completed a 12-week high monounsaturated fat, very low carbohydrate program.

The average weight loss was ~9.1 kg and the average waist measurement was reduced from ~117 to ~105 cm.

No adverse effects were recorded in any test. Subjects had a reduction in total cholesterol and triglycerides. HDL-C was unaffected.

Metabolic and Anthropometric changes in obese subjects from an unrestricted calorie, high monounsaturated fat, very low carbohydrate diet.
- 2000

5 endurance-trained cyclists participated in two 14-day randomized cross-over trials during which subjects consumed either their habitual diet or a high fat diet for 10 days, and then carb-loading for 3 days.

Subjects demonstrated an increased reliance on fat, a decreased reliance on muscle glycogen, and improved time trial performance after prolonged exercise.

High-fat diet versus habitual diet prior to carbohydrate loading: effects of exercise metabolism and cycling performance. - 2001

13 male untrained subjects were assigned either a high-fat or high carb diet, after 7 weeks of training and diet in fat-adapted subjects circulating fat in the blood appears to be an important substrate source during aerobic exercise, and in combination with the higher plasma fatty acid uptake it accounts for the increased fat oxidation observed during exercise.

Fat utilization during exercise: adaptation to a fat-rich diet increases utilization of plasma fatty acids and very low density lipoprotein-triglyceride in humans. - 2001

Testosterone, cortisol, and insulin responses to a high-fat test meal containing 1,300 kcal, 11% carbohydrate, 3% protein, 86% fat were determined before and after an 8-week high-fat diet (64% fat) in 11 healthy men.

The high-fat diet resulted in significant reductions in serum triglycerides.

There were no significant changes in testosterone and cortisol, but insulin concentrations were significantly lower at week 8.

After the fat-rich meal there were significant reductions for testosterone for 8 hours. Cortisol concentrations were significantly reduced 1 hour after the meal. Insulin was significantly increased at the 0-, 1-, and 2-hour postprandial time points before and after the high-fat diet.

Compared with week 0, insulin concentrations were significantly lower prior to and immediately after the fat-rich meal at week 8.

Effects of a high-fat diet on postabsorptive and postprandial testosterone responses to a fat-rich meal. - 2001

12 men switched from their habitual diet to a ketogenic diet and 8 control subjects consumed their habitual diet for 6 weeks.

There were significant decreases in fasting triglycerides, total and LDL cholesterol and oxidized LDL were unaffected, and HDL cholesterol tended to increase.

In subjects with a predominance of small LDL particles pattern B, there were significant increases in mean and peak LDL particle diameter and the percentage of LDL-1.

There were no significant changes in blood lipids in the

control group.

A Ketogenic Diet Favorably Affects Serum Biomarkers for Cardiovascular Disease in Normal-Weight Men. - 2002

7 cyclists underwent a 2-week adaptation to each of the following 3 diets: 14-day high carbohydrate; 14-day high fat; and 11.5-day high-fat diet followed by 2.5-day carbohydrate-loading.

Short term high-fat dietary conditioning increases fat oxidation and demonstrates evidence for enhanced ultra-endurance cycling performance, with little to no reduction in high output performance, relative to high-carbohydrate.

Effects of high-fat and high-carbohydrate diets on metabolism and performance in cycling. - 2002

6 healthy men were put on a eucaloric diet for a week of each a high-carbohydrate, ketogenic, and control diet.

The keto diet resulted in significantly lower glucose, insulin, and C-peptide. The fatty acid flux and whole-body fat oxidation were not affected by the high-carbohydrate diet compared with the control diet, but were increased by 67 and 47% respectively, on the ketogenic diet.

The effect of carbohydrate and fat variation in euenergetic diets on postabsorptive free fatty acid release. - 2002

41 overweight or obese people were placed on a very low carbohydrate diet with no limit on caloric intake for 6

months.

- mean body weight decreased ~10%
- total cholesterol level decreased
- LDL cholesterol level decreased
- triglyceride level decreased
- HDL cholesterol level increased
- cholesterol/HDL cholesterol ratio decreased

Effect of 6-month adherence to a very low carbohydrate diet program. - 2002

The effects of a very low carbohydrate diet were tested on fasting lipids, postprandial lipemia and markers of inflammation in women.

The diet modestly increased LDL-C, yet there were favorable effects on cardiovascular disease risk status by virtue of a relatively larger increase in HDL-C and a decrease in fasting and postprandial trigs.

An Isoenergetic Very Low Carbohydrate Diet Improves Serum HDL Cholesterol and triglyceride Concentrations, the Total Cholesterol to HDL Cholesterol Ratio and Postprandial Lipemic Responses Compared with a Low Fat Diet in Normal Weight, Normolipidemic Women. - 2003

18 children with autistic behavior were put on a ketogenic diet for 6 months, with continuous administration for 4 weeks, interrupted by 2-week diet-free intervals.

Significant improvement was recorded in 2 patients, average improvement in 8 patients, and minor improvement in 8 patients.

37 obese children were put on a diet of either ad-libitum very low carb or a low calorie balanced diet for 2 months.

Subjects in the very low carb group lost ~5.2kg whereas the subjects restricting calories actually gained ~2.4kg.

Effect of low-carbohydrate, unlimited calorie diet on the treatment of childhood obesity: a prospective controlled study. - 2003

80 elderly patients were put on a very low carbohydrate diet.

They experienced a reduction in:

- total cholesterol
- LDL cholesterol
- triglycerides
- LDL particle concentration
- small LDL
- and large VLDL

HDL cholesterol and large HDL increased.

Clinical use of a carbohydrate-restricted diet to treat the dyslipidemia of the metabolic syndrome. - 2003

11 duathletes ingested high-fat or high-carbohydrate diets for 5 weeks in a randomized crossover design.

Oxidative capacity in the muscles was not different after the 2 diet periods. Muscular fat stores significantly increased after high fat compared with high carb. Glycogen content was not significantly lower after high fat compared to carb.

Maximal power during an incremental exercise test to exhaustion, total work output during a 20-min all-out time trial, as well as half-marathon running time were not different between high fat and high carb.

Blood lactate concentrations and respiratory exchange ratios were significantly lower after high fat than high carb at rest and during all submaximal exercise loads.

Effects of dietary fat on muscle substrates, metabolism, and performance in athletes. - 2003

Obese non-diabetic patients with atherosclerotic cardiovascular disease who had previously been treated with statins were put on a high saturated fat, zero starch diet.

After 6 weeks the 23 patients had moderate decreases in bodyweight, fat percentage, triglycerides, VLDL trigs, size and concentration. HDL concentrations remained the same, but HDL and LDL size increased.

Some patients were monitored further on the same regime, 15 with polycystic ovary syndrome after 24 weeks lost ~14% bodyweight, and eight patients with reactive hypoglycemia after 52 weeks lost ~20% total bodyweight.

No subjects suffered adverse effects on serum lipids.

Effect of a high saturated fat and no-starch diet on serum lipid subfractions in patients with documented atherosclerotic cardiovascular disease. - 2003

13 healthy moderately overweight women were prescribed an energy restricted diet of either very low-carbohydrate or low-fat.

The low fat diet resulted in HDL-C significantly decreasing whilst fasting glucose, insulin, and insulin resistance were significantly increased. The very low-carbohydrate diet prevented decline in HDL-C and resulted in improved insulin sensitivity.

Comparison of a very low-carbohydrate and low-fat diet on fasting lipids, LDL subclasses, insulin resistance, and postprandial lipemic responses in overweight women. - 2004

28 healthy, overweight/obese men and women were prescribed 2 energy-restricted diets: ketogenic, or low fat with a goal similar to accepted recommendations.

Daily calories on the ketogenic diet for the men were ~1,855 compared to the ~1,562 on low fat. A distinct advantage of keto over low fat was demonstrated for weight loss, total fat loss, and trunk fat loss for men.

The majority of women also responded more favorably to the ketogenic diet, especially in terms of trunk fat loss.

Resting energy expenditure was decreased with both diets as expected, but was better maintained on the keto diet for men only. Individual responses clearly show the majority of men and women experience greater weight and fat loss on a low carb than a low fat diet.

Comparison of energy-restricted very low-carbohydrate and low-fat diets on weight loss and body composition in overweight men and women. -

96 insulin-resistant women were randomised to one of 3 dietary interventions: a high-carbohydrate high-fibre diet, a high-fat Atkins diet, or a high-protein Zone diet. There were supervised weight loss and weight maintenance phases (8 weeks each).

When compared with the high carb diet, the high fat and protein diets were shown to produce significantly greater reductions in weight, waist circumference, and triglycerides.

Comparison of high-fat and high-protein diets with a high-carbohydrate diet in insulin-resistant obese women. - 2005

In women with obesity and PCOS over a 24 week period, a ketogenic diet led to significant improvement in weight, percent free testosterone, LH/FSH ratio, and fasting insulin.

2 women became pregnant during the study despite previous infertility problems.

The effects of a low-carbohydrate, ketogenic diet on the polycystic ovary syndrome: a pilot study. - 2005

8 young, healthy volunteers ate a typical Western diet for 2 days, followed by 7 days of a low carb high protein diet.

This resulted in stimulated muscle protein synthesis

without gaining fat.

Effects of Dietary Carbohydrate Restriction with High Protein Intake on Protein Metabolism and the Somatotropic Axis. - 2005

21 overweight participants with type 2 diabetes maintained a ketogenic diet for 16-weeks.

- hemoglobin A1c decreased by ~16%
- diabetes medications were discontinued in 7 participants, reduced in 10 participants, and unchanged in 4 participants.
- body weight decreased by ~6.6%
- triglyceride decreased ~42%
- other serum lipid measurements did not change significantly

A low-carbohydrate, ketogenic diet to treat type 2 diabetes. - 2005

Obese patients with gastroesophageal reflux disease (GERD) were put on a very low carbohydrate diet, within 6 days outcomes included changes in the Johnson DeMeester score, percentage total time with a pH<4 in the distal esophagus, and GSAS-ds scores.

These data suggest that a very low-carbohydrate diet in obese individuals with GERD significantly reduces distal esophageal acid exposure and improves symptoms.

A Very Low-Carbohydrate Diet Improves Gastroesophageal Reflux and Its Symptoms. - 2006

People are concerned about low-carbohydrate ketogenic diets as they are said to increase bone turnover.

30 patients (15 study subjects and 15 controls) were assigned to either an unrestricted habitual diet or instructed to consume less than 20g of carbohydrates per day for the 1st month and then less than 40 g per day for months 2 and 3.

The keto dieters lost ~6.4kg versus ~1kg for the controls at 3 months, the diet did not increase bone turnover markers compared with controls at any time point.

The effect of a low-carbohydrate diet on bone turnover. - 2006

66 healthy obese subjects with BMI >30 with either normal or high cholesterol were put on a ketogenic diet for 56 weeks.

The body weight and body mass index decreased significantly. The level of total cholesterol, LDL cholesterol, triglycerides and blood glucose level decreased significantly, whereas HDL cholesterol increased significantly.

Long term effects of ketogenic diet in obese subjects with high cholesterol level. - 2006

59 subjects were put on a ketogenic diet with nutritional supplementation (including fish, borage and flaxseed oil).

The diet resulted in a significant shift from small, dense LDL to large, buoyant LDL.

5 patients with a BMI of ~36.4 and fatty liver disease were put on a ketogenic diet for 6 months.

Subjects lost ~13kg, and saw significant improvements of their fatty liver disease.

The Effect of a Low-Carbohydrate, Ketogenic Diet on Nonalcoholic Fatty Liver Disease: A Pilot Study. - 2007

Mood and other symptoms were evaluated by 119 overweight participants self-reporting whilst undergoing weight loss following either a ketogenic diet or a low-fat diet.

Self-reported symptom levels on seven scales were acquired: negative affect, fatigue, somatic symptoms, physical effects of hunger, insomnia, hunger, and stomach problems.

Participants experienced significant improvements in most symptoms regardless of diet. The keto group reported less negative affect and hunger, compared with the low fat group.

The effects of a low-carbohydrate ketogenic diet and a low-fat diet on mood, hunger, and other self-reported symptoms. - 2007

64 obese diabetic subjects were put on a ketogenic diet and monitored for 56 weeks, during which a significant

decrease in body weight, body mass index, the level of blood glucose, total cholesterol, LDL-cholesterol, triglycerides, and urea was expressed. The level of HDL-cholesterol increased significantly.

These changes were more significant in subjects with high blood glucose level as compared to those with normal blood glucose level.

The changes in the level of creatinine were not statistically significant.

Beneficial effects of ketogenic diet in obese diabetic subjects. - 2007

93 overweight or obese participants were randomly assigned to an energy-restricted low carb or low fat diet for 8 weeks.

There was some evidence for a smaller improvement in cognitive functioning with the LCHF diet with respect to speed of processing.

Low- and high-carbohydrate weight-loss diets have similar effects on mood but not cognitive performance. - 2007

Diabetic and non-diabetic subjects were randomly allocated to either a low-carbohydrate diet or a healthy-eating diet following Diabetes UK nutritional recommendations.

Weight loss was greater in the low-carbohydrate group, with no difference in changes in HbA1c, ketone or lipid levels.

The diet was equally effective in those with and without

diabetes.

A low-carbohydrate diet is more effective in reducing body weight than healthy eating in both diabetic and non-diabetic subjects. - 2007

88 obese adults were put on an either very low carb/high fat or high carb/low fat diet for 24 weeks, with energy restricted by 30%.

Weight loss was similar in both groups, the low carb group had greater decreases in triglycerides and increases in HDL cholesterol.

LDL cholesterol decreased in the high carb diet but remained unchanged in the low carb diet. However, a high degree of individual variability for the LDL response in the low carb diet. The apoB levels remained unchanged in both diet groups.

Metabolic Effects of Weight Loss on a Very-Low-Carbohydrate Diet Compared With an Isocaloric High-Carbohydrate Diet in Abdominally Obese Subjects. - 2008

Obese children between 6 and 12 years old were put on a diet restricted in carbs to <30g but otherwise unrestricted in fat and protein.

Cholesterol and triglycerides were reduced significantly after 10 weeks.

Unlimited energy, restricted carbohydrate diet improves lipid parameters in obese children - 2008

The effect of a very-low-carbohydrate, high-saturated-fat diet on markers of endothelial function and cardiovascular disease risk was compared with that of an isocaloric high-carbohydrate, low-saturated-fat diet.

Weight loss occurred in both groups and was significantly greater in the low carb group, BMI also decreased, with a differential effect of diet such that the reduction was greater in the low carb group.

HDL cholesterol did not change with the high carb group, but increased with low carb. Triglycerides decreased overall, to a greater extent with the low carb diet.

A very-low-carbohydrate high fat diet with significant portion as saturated fat diet not impair brachial artery flow-mediated dilatation.

Effects of weight loss from a very-low-carbohydrate diet on endothelial function and markers of cardiovascular disease risk in subjects with abdominal obesity. - 2008

This Ketogenic diet was called "Spanish Ketogenic Mediterranean Diet" (SKMD) due to the incorporation of virgin olive oil as the principal source of fat, moderate red wine intake, green vegetables and salads as the main source of carbohydrates, and fish as the main source of proteins. It was an unlimited calorie diet.

31 obese subjects around 40 years old undertook the regimen for 3 months.

There was a significant reduction in:

- body weight (~14kg)
- BMI (~5pts)
- systolic and diastolic blood pressure

- total cholesterol (~208 → ~186)
- triacylglicerols (~halved)
- glucose (~110 → ~93)
- LDL-C (~114 → ~106)

HDL-C saw an increase.

Spanish Ketogenic Mediterranean diet: a healthy cardiovascular diet for weight loss. - 2008

31 healthy people of age ~52 were on a low carb high fat diet for at least 1 year, most more than 3 years, with an average of 4 years adherence.

The longer the adherence to the diet the lower the blood pressure and BMI.

Averages for total cholesterol were ~270, LDL-C ~180, HDL-C ~70, triglycerides ~93, and the trig:HDL ratio 1.4. Insulin resistance was very low.

In most subjects glucose, insulin, glucagon, cortisol, homocysteine, glycerol, and C-reactive protein were within reference ranges.

Long-term consumption of a carbohydrate-restricted diet does not induce deleterious metabolic effects. - 2008

119 overweight subjects were randomized to follow a ketogenic diet or a low-fat diet for 24 weeks.

Mental aspects of health-related quality of life improved more in participants following a ketogenic diet than a low fat diet, possibly resulting from the keto diet's composition, lack of energy restriction, higher levels of satiety, or metabolic effects.

Effects of two weight-loss diets on health-related quality of life. - 2009

This case study follows a 70 year old woman diagnosed with schizophrenia, paranoia, disorganized speech, and hallucinations, including seeing skeletons and hearing voices that told her to hurt herself, since childhood.

A typical day's diet was egg and cheese sandwiches, diet soda, water, pimento cheese, barbequed pork, chicken salad, hamburger helper, macaroni and cheese, and potatoes.

She was put on a ketogenic diet consisting of unlimited meats and eggs, 4 ounces of hard cheese, 2 cups of salad vegetables, and 1 cup of low-carbohydrate vegetables per day.

After just over a week she was no longer hearing voices or seeing skeletons, there was no change in medication.

After 12 months she had no recurrence of hallucinations, had lost ~10kg, and experienced improvements in energy level.

Even with 2–3 isolated episodes of dietary non-compliance that lasted several days where she ate pasta, bread, and cakes, there was no recurrence of hallucinations.

Schizophrenia, gluten, and low-carbohydrate, ketogenic diets: a case report and review of the literature. - 2009

60 subjects with BMI ~33 were randomly assigned to an

energy restricted low or high carb diet for 8 weeks.

The low carb diet shifted fuel utilization toward greater fat oxidation during exercise, but had no detrimental effect on high intensity or endurance aerobic exercise performance or muscle strength compared with a high carb diet.

Effects of a low carbohydrate weight loss diet on exercise capacity and tolerance in obese subjects. - 2009

13 participants with moderate to severe IBS-D completed a 2-week standard diet, then 4 weeks of a very low carbohydrate diet.

77% reported adequate relief for all 4 low carb weeks. Stool frequency decreased, stool consistency improved, abdominal pain scores and quality-of-life measures significantly improved.

A Very Low-Carbohydrate Diet Improves Symptoms and Quality of Life in Diarrhea-Predominant Irritable Bowel Syndrome. - 2009

A frequently cited concern of very-low-carbohydrate diets is the potential for increased risk of kidney disease associated with a higher protein intake.

68 obese subjects without preexisting renal dysfunction were randomized to consume either an energy-restricted very-low-carbohydrate or high-carbohydrate diet.

By 1 year, there were no changes in either group in serum creatinine levels, providing preliminary evidence that long-term weight loss with a very-low-carbohydrate diet does not adversely affect renal function compared with a high-carbohydrate diet in obese individuals with normal kidney function.

Renal function following long-term weight loss in individuals with abdominal obesity on a very-low-carbohydrate diet vs high-carbohydrate diet. - 2010

A 65-year-old woman with brain cancer was put on a calorie restricted ketogenic diet as well as given standard therapy.

After 2 months treatment, the patient's body weight was reduced by about 20% and no discernable brain tumor tissue was detected, biomarker changes showed reduced levels of blood glucose and elevated levels of urinary ketones.

10 weeks after suspension of strict diet therapy MRI evidence of tumor recurrence was found.

Metabolic management of glioblastoma multiforme using standard therapy together with a restricted ketogenic diet: Case Report. - 2010

The ketogenic diet has well-established short- and long-term outcomes for children with intractable epilepsy, in this study there were many subjects who were once patients contacted to understand the long-term effects.

Results demonstrate that even after discontinuation, the majority of subjects are still doing well with regard to health and seizure control.

Long-term outcomes of children treated with the ketogenic diet in the past. - 2010

Severely obese adolescents were put on a high protein, low carbohydrate regimen for 13 weeks, with follow-up at 36 weeks.

Significant reduction in BMI was achieved during intervention, and maintained at follow-up.

The high protein low carbohydrate diet is a safe and effective option for medically supervised weight loss in severely obese adolescents.

Efficacy and Safety of a High Protein, Low Carbohydrate Diet for Weight Loss in Severely Obese Adolescents. - 2010

Obese subjects without diabetes or dyslipidemia were put on either an unlimited calorie low-carbohydrate diet or low-fat diet of limited energy intake (1200-1800kcal or <30% fat). Low carbers were at 20g/d for 3 months and then increased carbohydrate intake 5g/d per wk until a stable and desired weight was achieved.

During the first 6 months the low-carbohydrate diet group had greater reductions in diastolic blood pressure, triglyceride levels, and VLDL cholesterol levels, lesser reductions in LDL cholesterol levels, and greater increases in HDL cholesterol levels at all time points.

Weight and metabolic outcomes after 2 years on a low-carbohydrate versus low-fat diet: a randomized trial. - 2010

22 obese subjects with metabolic syndrome were assigned a Spanish Ketogenic Mediterranean Diet for 12 weeks.

There was an extremely significant improvement in LDL

cholesterol and all the parameters studied associated with metabolic syndrome: body weight down ~15kg, BMI down ~5, waist circumference down ~17cm, fasting glucose down ~25, triglycerides halved, HDL cholesterol up ~25%, blood pressure significantly reduced.

After the diet all the subjects were free of metabolic syndrome according to the International Diabetes Federation definition, and 100% of them had normal triglycerides and HDL cholesterol levels, in spite of the fact that most of them still had a BMI > 30.

A pilot study of the Spanish Ketogenic Mediterranean Diet: an effective therapy for the metabolic syndrome. 2011

14 obese men with non-alcoholic fatty liver disease were put on the "Spanish Ketogenic Mediterranean Diet" for 12 weeks.

- significant loss of body weight
- improvement in LDL-cholesterol
- ~21% of subjects saw complete fatty liver regression
- ~93% of subjects saw overall reduction in liver disease
- all biomarkers of metabolic syndrome improved significantly: BMI, waist circumference, fasting plasma glucose, triglycerides, HDL-cholesterol, systolic blood pressure, and diastolic blood pressure

The effect of the Spanish Ketogenic Mediterranean Diet on nonalcoholic fatty liver disease: a pilot study - 2011

Obese adults were randomly assigned to a low carb or

low fat diet for 2 years. Cravings for specific types of foods (sweets, high-fats, fast-food fats, and carbohydrates/starches); preferences for high-sugar, high-carbohydrate, and low-carbohydrate/high-protein foods; and appetite were measured.

The low carb diet had significantly larger decreases in cravings for carbohydrates/starches and high-sugar foods, and reported being less bothered by hunger, and that men had larger reductions in appetite compared to women.

Change in food cravings, food preferences, and appetite during a low-carbohydrate and low-fat diet. - 2011

106 subjects with a BMI ≥ 25 were put on a modified ketogenic diet based on green vegetables, olive oil, fish and meat plus dishes composed of high quality protein and virtually zero carbohydrate, with the addition of some herbal extracts. Calories in the diet were unlimited.

After 6 weeks there was a significant reduction in BMI and weight, fat mass percentage, waist circumference, total cholesterol, LDL-C, triglycerides, and blood glucose. HDL-C increased significantly.

There were no significant changes in BUN, ALT, AST, GGT and blood creatinine.

Effect of ketogenic mediterranean diet with phytoextracts and low carbohydrates/high-protein meals on weight, cardiovascular risk factors, body composition and diet compliance in Italian council employees. - 2011

58 obese children were placed on either a ketogenic or

low calorie diet for 6 months.

The ketogenic diet revealed more pronounced improvements in weight loss and metabolic parameters than the hypocaloric diet.

Metabolic impact of a ketogenic diet compared to a hypocaloric diet in obese children and adolescents. - 2012

307 obese adults without serious medical illnesses were randomly assigned to a low-carbohydrate high-protein or a low-fat weight-loss diet for 24 months.

There was no noticeably harmful effects on kidney function, albuminuria, or fluid and electrolyte balance compared with a low-fat diet.

Comparative effects of low-carbohydrate high-protein versus low-fat diets on the kidney. - 2012

Subjects were put on a 20 day ketogenic or a low-calorie Mediterranean diet.

Both diet protocols lead to a significant decrease in body weight, the reduction was significantly greater on keto. The ketogenic diet also lead to increased fat oxidation at rest without any effect on resting energy expenditure. Interestingly this effect was long lasting, at least for up to 20 days following cessation of the ketogenic diet.

Medium term effects of a ketogenic diet and a Mediterranean diet on resting energy expenditure and respiratory ratio. - 2012

8 athletes were analyzed for body composition and various performance aspects before and after 30 days of a modified ketogenic diet. The diet was based on green vegetables, olive oil, fish and meat plus dishes composed of high quality protein and virtually zero carbohydrates.

No significant differences were detected between the ketogenic and standard diet in all strength tests. Significant differences were found in body weight and body composition: after keto there was a decrease in body weight and fat mass with a non-significant increase in muscle mass.

Ketogenic diet does not affect strength performance in elite artistic gymnasts. - 2012

Patients with advanced incurable cancers, normal organ function without diabetes or recent weight loss, and a body mass index of at least 20, were put on a ketogenic diet.

Preliminary data demonstrate that an insulin-inhibiting ketogenic diet is safe and feasible in selected patients with advanced cancer. The extent of ketosis, but not calorie deficit or weight loss, correlated with stable disease or partial remission.

Targeting insulin inhibition as a metabolic therapy in advanced cancer: a pilot safety and feasibility dietary trial in 10 patients. - 2012

Reduced resting and total energy expenditure (REE / TEE) following weight loss is thought to contribute to the prevalence of weight regain after dieting and then resuming a normal diet.

21 overweight young adults were put on a weight loss diet, after achieving 10-15% weight loss they were put on a weight maintenance diet of the same calories, but consisting of either low-fat, low-glycemic index, or very low-carbohydrate. This was done in a controlled 3-way crossover design in random order, each for 4 weeks.

Compared with the pre-weight-loss baseline, the decrease in REE and TEE was greatest with the low-fat diet, intermediate with the low-glycemic index diet, and least with the very low-carbohydrate diet, meaning the low-fat diet caused as much as a 300 calorie drop in expenditure despite the same intake and activity levels as the low carb diet.

Effects of dietary composition on energy expenditure during weight-loss maintenance. - 2012

363 overweight and obese people were put on a 24 week diet intervention trial, free to choose either a low calorie or ketogenic diet.

Both diets had beneficial effects on all the parameters: body weight, BMI, waist circumference, blood glucose level, HbA1c, total cholesterol, LDL-C, HDL-C, triglycerides, uric acid, urea and creatinine.

These changes were more significant in subjects who were on the ketogenic diet as compared with those restricting calories.

Effect of low-calorie versus low-carbohydrate ketogenic diet in type 2 diabetes. - 2012

22 healthy subjects received a ketogenic zero carb diet or 55% carbohydrate diet of equal calories in a randomised cross-over design.

During the zero carb diet gluconeogenesis was increased, glucose was lower, ketone bodies were significantly higher, and appetite was suppressed.

Gluconeogenesis and protein-induced satiety. - 2012

2 women with type II bipolar disorder were able to maintain ketosis for prolonged periods of time (2 and 3 years, respectively). Both experienced mood stabilization that exceeded that achieved with medication; experienced a significant subjective improvement that was distinctly related to ketosis; and tolerated the diet well. There were no significant adverse effects in either case.

One reported her diet as diverse with meats (organic grass fed beef, organic pork, and free-range chickens), dairy products (raw whole milk, cream, cheeses), and seafood (salt water fish, clams, shrimp).

The other commented "I find the diet very palatable, and easy to follow. I eat a lot of fish (sardines, salmon, tuna), olive oil, coconut milk, butter, fatty meat, eggs, some bacon, poultry with skin, and some nuts. I use 1–2 tablespoons of coconut oil if I happen to have a few more carbs on any particular day, as this keeps me ketogenic. I have about 1–2 cups of veggies as my daily carb source."

Results suggest that a ketogenic diet can act as a mood stabilizer in patients with type II bipolar disorder.

The ketogenic diet for type II bipolar disorder. - 2013

Subjects with strength training experience performed a variety of tests after a week of a habitual moderate carb diet (~2,530 cals) then again after a week on a very low carb diet (~2,150 cals).

Body mass decreased significantly, despite this, strength and power outputs were maintained for both men and women.

Effects of a short-term carbohydrate-restricted diet on strength and power performance. - 2013

Migraine sufferers were assigned either a standard or ketogenic diet, after one month headache frequency and drug consumption was reduced in the keto group.

Responder rates were higher than 90% in terms of attack frequency and drug consumption.

Short term improvement of migraine headaches during ketogenic diet: a prospective observational study in a dietician clinical setting. - 2013

The circulating concentrations of several hormones and nutrients which influence appetite were altered after weight loss induced by a ketogenic diet, compared with after refeeding.

39 subjects completed an 8-week ketogenic restricted energy diet, followed by 2 weeks of reintroduction of foods. When participants were ketotic, the weight loss induced increase in ghrelin was suppressed. Subjective ratings of appetite were lower at week 8 than after refeeding.

Ketosis and appetite-mediating nutrients and hormones after weight loss. -

This meta-analysis aimed to investigate whether individuals assigned to a ketogenic diet achieve better long-term body weight and cardiovascular risk factor management when compared with individuals assigned to a conventional low-fat diet.

5 outcomes revealed significant results. Individuals assigned to keto showed decreased body weight, triglycerides, and diastolic blood pressure, while increased HDL-C and LDL-C.

Individuals assigned to a ketogenic diet achieve a greater weight loss than those assigned to a low fat diet in the long-term.

Very-low-carbohydrate ketogenic diet v. low-fat diet for long-term weight loss: a meta-analysis of randomised controlled trials. - 2013

Advanced glycation end products (AGEs) are substances formed by glycation which in simple terms is much like cells/proteins becoming glued together, and can be a factor in the development or worsening of many degenerative diseases, such as diabetes, atherosclerosis, chronic renal failure and Alzheimer's disease. Also heavily implicated in age-related degeneration and diseases, oxidative stress on cells and LDL particles, arterial stiffness, and the list goes on.

In this study, the inhibitory effect of ketone bodies on AGEs formation was studied after 35 days of incubation. The measurements of glycated HSA by glucose in the presence of ketones indicates a decrease in AGEs formation.

The concentration of ketones used in this study is in accordance with the concentration detected in the body of individuals post fasting and prolonged exercises, or on a ketogenic diet.

Inhibition of fluorescent advanced glycation end products (AGEs) of human serum albumin upon incubation with 3-β-hydroxybutyrate. - 2014

Subjects were assigned to either a medium carb/low fat/calorie restricted (MCCR) diet as specified by the American Diabetes Association, or an unrestricted ketogenic diet.

After 3 months HbA1c level was unchanged in the MCCR diet group, while it decreased in the keto group. 44% of the keto subjects discontinued one or more diabetes medications, compared to 11% of the MCCR group.

The keto group lost more weight, ~5.5kg vs ~2.6kg.

A Randomized Pilot Trial of a Moderate Carbohydrate Diet Compared to a Very Low Carbohydrate Diet in Overweight or Obese Individuals with Type 2 Diabetes Mellitus or Prediabetes. - 2014

General Carbohydrate Restriction and Ketosis

28 patients with chronic migraine problems were put on a ketogenic diet. Some patients had poor compliance, however 9 reported some improvement.

An Experience with a Ketogenic Dietary in Migraine - 1928

2 healthy men lived exclusively for 1 year on lean and fat meat, 120-130 grams of protein and enough fat to make a total intake of 2600 to 3000 calories per day.

During the consumption of large quantities of fat ketonuria was present, at no time was ketoacidosis demonstrated.

Urine analysis and other tests for renal function revealed no abnormalities.

The blood was little affected, except for minor elevated fat and cholesterol.

Uric acid levels rose but returned to normal after a few months whilst still on the diet.

The Effect of an Exclusive Meat Diet on the Chemical Constituents of the Blood. - 1929

Restriction of carbohydrate, alone, appears to make possible the treatment of obesity on a calorically unrestricted diet composed chiefly of protein and fat. The limiting factor on appetite, necessary to any treatment of obesity, appears to be provided by increased mobilisation and utilisation of fat, in conjunction with the homeostatic forces which normally regulate the appetite.

Ketogenesis appears to be a key factor in the increased utilisation of fat.

Treatment of obesity by this method appears to avoid the decline in the metabolism encountered in treatment by caloric restriction.

Treatment of OBESITY with Calorically UNRESTRICTED DIETS. - 1953

5 obese women were fed 400 calories from single energy sources and 800 calorie combinations of these.

At 400 calories a day, ketosis was least with carbohydrate and greatest with fat as the diet, as protein ketosis was reduced.

The addition of 400 calories of carbohydrate to 400 calories of protein was found to effectively prevent the development of ketosis, addition as fat did not.

Loss of weight, sodium, and potassium was much greater with diets based on fat than on carbohydrate.

Ketosis, weight loss, uric acid, and nitrogen balance in obese women fed single nutrients at low caloric levels - 1969

A group of obese men with no significant blood ketones injected with insulin suffered clinical signs of hypoglycaemia (sweating, nervousness, tachycardia, rising blood pressure, constricting chest pain, and mental confusion) as their blood glucose levels dropped from

~5.5 to under ~3.0.

After 2 months of fasting the subjects had lost ~33kg, their blood glucose levels were ~4.5, and ketone levels were around ~8.0. After a follow-up round of insulin shots the subjects blood glucose levels plummeted to ~2.0 - enough to result in a coma for a normal-fed person - but they suffered no ill consequences of low blood sugar or any particular reactions to the insulin.

Resistance to symptomatic insulin reactions after fasting. - 1972

Ketone bodies accumulate in the plasma in conditions of fasting and uncontrolled diabetes. The initiating event is a change in the ratio of glucagon:insulin.

Low insulin levels trigger breakdown in adipose tissue with the result that free fatty acids pass into the plasma for uptake by liver and other tissues. Glucagon appears to be the primary hormone involved in the induction of fatty acid oxidation and ketogenesis in the liver.

Administration of food after a fast, or of insulin to the diabetic subject, reduces plasma free fatty acid concentrations, increases the liver concentration of malonyl-CoA, inhibits carnitine acyltransferase I and reverses the ketogenic process.

The regulation of ketogenesis. - 1982

During a ketogenic regimen concentrations of fat derived substrates rise significantly and glucose levels decrease, hormonal patterns switch towards a catabolic mode with a fall in insulin levels and a rise in glucagon concentration, levels of gluconeogenic amino acids are reduced while those of the branched chain amino acids increase.

These changes also reproduce those observed after a few days of total fasting, suggesting it is the carbohydrate restriction itself which is responsible.

Hormonal and metabolic changes induced by an isocaloric isoproteinic ketogenic diet in healthy subjects. - 1982

Post-exercise ketosis was first described in 1909 by Forssner, who found that his daily excretion of acetone in the urine was increased on days when he had undertaken a brisk walk in the morning.

Athletes on unrestricted diets eat more, particularly carbohydrates, than non-athletes, and have lower post-exercise ketone body levels. They also have lower plasma glucagon, growth hormone, catecholamine, and free-fatty acid levels during sub-maximal exercise.

On a standard ~2,800 calorie diet, however, non-athletes have the lower post-exercise ketone body levels. The hormone response of athletes and non-athletes to exercise can similarly be reversed by dietary manipulation.

The carbohydrate status of the body is, therefore, probably the main determinant of the type of blood hormone profile that develops during exercise, and the degree of ketosis that develops after exercise.

Post-exercise ketosis and the hormone response to exercise: a review. - 1982

Elevation of ketones may offer neuroprotection in the

treatment or prevention of both Alzheimer's disease, where therapy is lacking, and Parkinson's disease, where therapy with L-dopa is time limited.

d-β-Hydroxybutyrate protects neurons in models of Alzheimer's and Parkinson's disease - 2000

A retrospective review of 32 infants who had been treated with the ketogenic diet were able to maintain strong ketosis. The overall effectiveness of the diet in infants was similar to that reported in the literature for older children.

The diet was particularly effective for patients with infantile spasms/myoclonic seizures. There were concomitant reductions in antiepileptic medications. The majority of parents reported improvements in seizure frequency and in their child's behavior and function, particularly with respect to attention/alertness, activity level, and socialization.

The diet generally was well-tolerated, and 96.4% maintained appropriate growth parameters.

Experience with the ketogenic diet in infants. - 2001

Ketosis has been central to starving man's survival by providing nonglucose substrate to his evolutionarily hypertrophied brain, sparing muscle from destruction for glucose synthesis.

Ketone bodies may also provide a more efficient source of energy for brain per unit of oxygen, it has also been shown to decrease cell death in 2 human neuronal cultures, one a model of Alzheimer's and the other of Parkinson's disease.

The ability of ketone bodies to oxidize co-enzyme Q and reduce NADP+ may also be important in decreasing free radical damage.

Ketone bodies, potential therapeutic uses. - 2001

In testing subjects ability to enter a "good" level of ketosis with or without prior fasting, mean time to onset of ketosis was 33 hours and to good ketosis, 58 hours. The ketogenic diet can be effectively initiated without a fast.

Is a fast necessary when initiating the ketogenic diet? - 2002

Breath acetone is as good a predictor of ketosis as is urinary acetoacetate. Breath acetone analysis is noninvasive and can be performed frequently with minimal discomfort to patients.

Breath acetone is a reliable indicator of ketosis in adults consuming ketogenic meals. - 2002

Since the metabolism of ketone bodies is thermodynamically more efficient than the metabolism of glucose, a shift in brain energy metabolism from glucose to ketones will produce a homeostatic state that is capable of restoring the physiological balance of excitation and inhibition.

Ketones displace glucose as the predominating fuel for the brain, decreasing the need for glucose synthesis and accordingly spares its precursor, muscle-derived amino acids.

Without this metabolic adaptation, H. sapiens could not have evolved such a large brain.

Ketones are not just a fuel, but a "superfuel" more efficiently producing ATP energy than glucose or fatty acid.

Ketoacids? Good medicine? - 2003

Normal mammalian brain cells are metabolically versatile and capable of deriving energy from glucose and ketone bodies. Ketone bodies bypass the glucose-based pathway which causes significant increases in metabolites and improves physiological performance through an increase in the energy generated.

Ketone body metabolism reduces oxygen free radicals, enhances tolerance to hypoxia (limited oxygen), and may prevent organ dysfunction from inflammatory processes.

A shift in energy metabolism from glucose to ketones will enhance the storage and use of energy of normal brain cells.

Role of glucose and ketone bodies in the metabolic control of experimental brain cancer. - 2003

Until recently, ketosis was viewed with apprehension in the medical world; however, current advances in nutritional research have discounted this apprehension and increased public awareness about its favourable effects.

One argument against the consumption of a high fat diet is that it causes obesity. Because fat has a higher caloric density than carbohydrate, it is thought that the consumption of a high fat diet will be accompanied by a higher energy intake. On the contrary, recent studies have observed that a ketogenic diet can be used as a therapy for weight reduction in obese patients.

It has been found that a sugary diet is the root cause of various chronic diseases of the body. Several recent studies have pointed to the fact that a diet with a high glycemic load is independently associated with the development of cardiovascular diseases, type II diabetes and certain forms of cancer.

It has been shown that short-term ketogenic diets improve the lipid disorders that are characteristic of atherogenic dyslipidemia (elevated trigs, small LDL particles, and reduced HDL-C).

Sugar consumption is positively associated with cancer in humans and test animals. It has also been found that the risk of breast cancer decreases with increases in total fat intake.

Long-term effects of a ketogenic diet in obese patients. - 2004

In comparison with glucose, ketone bodies are actually a very good respiratory fuel.

Indeed, there is no clear requirement for dietary

carbohydrates for human adults.

Contrary to popular belief, insulin is not needed for glucose uptake and utilization in man.

Low-carbohydrate diets have been avoided because of the high-fat nature of the diets and the "predicted" associated hypercholesterolemia. However, serum lipids generally improve with the low-carbohydrate diet, especially the triglyceride and HDL measurements.

Replacement of fat with carbohydrates however results in significant reductions in HDL cholesterol.

Metabolic Effects of the Very-Low-Carbohydrate Diets: Misunderstood "Villains" of Human Metabolism. - 2004

The effects of ketone body metabolism suggests that mild ketosis may offer therapeutic potential in a variety of different common and rare disease states.

The large categories of disease for which ketones may have therapeutic effects are:

1. diseases of substrate insufficiency or insulin resistance,
2. diseases resulting from free radical damage,
3. disease resulting from hypoxia.

The therapeutic implications of ketone bodies: the effects of ketone bodies in pathological conditions: ketosis, ketogenic diet, redox states, insulin resistance, and mitochondrial metabolism - 2004

In Alzheimer's disease (AD), there appears to be a pathological decrease in the brain's ability to use glucose.

Neurobiological evidence suggests that ketone bodies are an effective alternative energy substrate for the brain.

Elevation of plasma ketone body levels through an oral dose of medium chain triglycerides may improve cognitive functioning in older adults with memory disorders. Higher ketone values were associated with greater improvement in paragraph recall with MCT treatment.

Effects of β-hydroxybutyrate on cognition in memory-impaired adults. - 2004

Impaired physical performance is a common but not obligate result of a short-term low carbohydrate diet.

Until the development of agriculture over last few millennia, consumption of dietary carbohydrate was opportunistic. Fat and protein were the primary sources of dietary energy.

Time for adaptation, optimized sodium and potassium intake, and constraint of protein to 15–25 % of daily energy expenditure allow unimpaired endurance performance despite nutritional ketosis.

Ketogenic diets and physical performance. - 2004

Very low-carbohydrate diets (VLCDs) are popular, but remain controversial.

This review summarizes the latest studies that have examined the effects of VLCDs on lipoproteins and related risk factors for cardiovascular disease.

Prospective studies indicate that VLCDs improve the

lipoprotein profile independently of weight loss.

VLCDs consistently improve postabsorptive and postprandial triglycerides, HDL cholesterol, and the distribution of LDL-C subfractions to a greater extent than low-fat diets.

VLCDs also improve proinflammatory markers when associated with weight loss.

Considering the effectiveness of VLCDs in promoting fat loss and improving the metabolic syndrome, discounting or condemning their use is unjustified.

Modification of Lipoproteins by Very Low-Carbohydrate Diets. - 2005

Urinary and serum ketones are detected during low-carbohydrate diets, however it's not an obligate indicator of weight loss.

Urinary ketones reflect serum ketone concentration but do not relate to weight loss in overweight premenopausal women following a low-carbohydrate/high-protein diet. - 2005

Due to its use by brain, ketone bodies not only permit man to survive prolonged starvation, but also may have therapeutic potential owing to its greater efficiency in providing cellular energy in blood restricted states such as stroke, myocardial insufficiency, neonatal stress, genetic mitochondrial problems, and physical fatigue.

Fuel metabolism in starvation. - 2006

Altering the macronutrient composition of the diet influences hunger and satiety. Studies have compared high- and low-protein diets, but there are few data on carbohydrate content and ketosis on motivation to eat and ad libitum intake.

In the short term, high-protein, low-carbohydrate ketogenic diets reduce hunger and lower food intake significantly more than do high-protein, medium-carbohydrate nonketogenic diets.

Effects of a high-protein ketogenic diet on hunger, appetite, and weight loss in obese men feeding ad libitum. - 2008

An early feature of Alzheimer's disease is region-specific declines in brain glucose metabolism. Inhibition of glucose metabolism can have profound effects on brain function.

One promising approach is to supplement the normal glucose supply of the brain with ketone bodies. Much of the benefit of ketone bodies can be attributed to their ability to increase mitochondrial efficiency and supplement the brain's normal reliance on glucose.

Ketone bodies as a therapeutic for Alzheimer's disease. - 2008

The ketogenic diet up-regulates glutathione biosynthesis, enhances mitochondrial antioxidant status, and protects mtDNA from oxidant-induced damage.

The ketogenic diet increases mitochondrial glutathione levels - 2008

As well as the weight loss, ketogenic diets promote a non-atherogenic lipid profile, lower blood pressure, and diminish resistance to insulin with an improvement in blood levels of glucose and insulin.

Such diets also have anti-tumor benefits, do not alter renal or liver functions, do not produce metabolic acidosis by ketosis, have many neurological benefits in the central nervous system, do not produce osteoporosis and could increase the performance in aerobic sports.

Ketogenic diets: additional benefits to the weight loss and unfounded secondary effects - 2008

Parents and neurologists were sometimes reluctant to start children on the traditional ketogenic diet, the modified Atkins diet (MAD) was created at Johns Hopkins Hospital as an attempt to create a more palatable and less restrictive dietary treatment primarily for children with behavioral difficulties.

The MAD was designed to mimic ketosis while providing similar but unlimited quantities of high fat (and protein) foods, and has been reported as efficacious as a traditional ketogenic diet in eight publications to date by centers in four countries.

The diet is "modified" from the Atkins diet as the "induction phase" of the diet limiting carbohydrates is maintained indefinitely, fat is encouraged (not just allowed), and weight loss is not the goal (unless nutritionally indicated).

At the time of the writing of this review, there have been 100 reported children and adults started on the diet, 45% have had 50–90% seizure reduction, and 28% >90% seizure reduction.

Brain tumors are potentially manageable with dietary therapies that lower glucose availability and elevate ketone bodies. These diets target tumor energy metabolism and reduce tumor growth through integrated anti-inflammatory, antiangiogenic, and proapoptotic mechanisms of action.

Targeting energy metabolism in brain cancer with calorically restricted ketogenic diets. - 2008

A characteristic of Alzheimer's disease is regional hypometabolism in the brain. This decline in cerebral glucose metabolism occurs before pathology and symptoms manifest, continues as symptoms progress, and is more severe than that of normal aging.

Ketone bodies are an efficient alternative fuel for cells that are unable to metabolize glucose or are 'starved' of glucose.

Hypometabolism as a therapeutic target in Alzheimer's disease. - 2008

Seven aggressive human cancer cell lines, and 3 control fibroblast lines were grown in vitro in either glucose, or in glucose plus ketone bodies.

Controls demonstrated normal cell growth, while all cancer lines in ketone bodies demonstrated proportionally inhibited growth.

The results bear on the hypothesized potential for ketogenic diets as therapeutic strategies.

Acetoacetate reduces growth and ATP concentration in cancer cell lines which over-express uncoupling protein 2. - 2009

An expanding body of evidence indicates that ketone bodies are indeed neuroprotective.

Ketone bodies protect neurons against multiple types of neuronal injury and the underlying mechanisms are similar to those of calorie restriction and of the ketogenic diet.

THE NEUROPROTECTIVE PROPERTIES OF CALORIE RESTRICTION, THE KETOGENIC DIET, AND KETONE BODIES. - 2009

As primarily a metabolic disease, malignant brain cancer can be managed through changes in metabolic environment. In contrast to normal neurons and glia, which readily transition to ketone bodies for energy under reduced glucose, malignant brain tumors are strongly dependent on glucose for energy.

This approach to brain cancer management is supported from recent studies in mice and humans treated with calorie restriction and the ketogenic diet.

Metabolic management of brain cancer. - 2011

Since its introduction in 1921, the ketogenic diet has been in continuous use for children with difficult-to-control epilepsy.

After decades of relative disuse, it is now both extremely popular and well studied, future non-epilepsy indications such as Alzheimer disease, amyotrophic lateral sclerosis (Lou Gehrig's disease), autism, and brain tumors are under active investigation.

Dietary treatment of epilepsy: rebirth of an ancient treatment. - 2011

Data supporting the hypothesis that insulin can be a pathogenic contributor to acne also come from the observations of increased acne in women with polycystic ovary syndrome (PCOS) which is a condition associated with increased insulin resistance and hyperinsulinemia.

The evidence suggests that the ketogenic diet could be an effective therapeutic tool in the hands of the health care professional for a reduction acne as well as diseases that may be associated with it.

Ketosis reduces several markers of inflammation, reducing insulinemia, which also affects the IGF-1 pathway, it could be effective in reducing the severity and progression of acne.

Nutrition and Acne: Therapeutic Potential of Ketogenic Diets. - 2012

The ketogenic diet has a wide range of neurological effects, the following are just some of the spectrum of observations of ketone bodies thus far which require further research:

- raise ATP levels and reduce ROS production, demonstrating neuroprotective properties
- stimulate mitochondrial biogenesis

- stabilise synaptic function
- reduces glycolysis, which suppresses seizures and prolongs lifespan of numerous species
- aged rats have significantly increased mitochondrial density and cerebral function, problem solving and recognition performance
- protect against the toxic effects of ß-amyloid on neurons in culture
- mice benefit from better mitochondrial function, less oxidative stress, and reduced expression of amyloid precursor protein and ß-amyloid
- mitochondrial respiratory chain damage from a toxin is ameliorated in mice
- animals with brain tumors exhibit markedly decreased tumor growth rates
- reductions in ROS production in malignant glioma cells
- rats with induced cardiac arrest and stroke found significantly reduced neurodegeneration
- cognitive and motor functioning are improved
- tissue sparing in brain following injury
- autistic children demonstrate moderate or significant behavioral improvement
- significant reduction in the velocity of cortical spreading depression velocity in immature rats

The ketogenic diet as a treatment paradigm for diverse neurological disorders. - 2012

Very-low-carbohydrate ketogenic diets have been in use since the 1920s as a therapy for epilepsy and can, in some cases, completely remove the need for medication.

From the 1960s onwards they have become widely known as one of the most common methods for obesity treatment.

Recent work over the last decade or so has provided evidence of the therapeutic potential of ketogenic diets in many pathological conditions, such as diabetes, polycystic ovary syndrome, acne, neurological diseases, cancer and the amelioration of respiratory and cardiovascular disease risk factors.

Beyond weight loss: a review of the therapeutic uses of very-low-carbohydrate (ketogenic) diets. - 2013

Accumulating evidence suggests that low-carbohydrate, high-fat diets are safe and effective to reduce glycemia in diabetic patients without producing significant cardiovascular risks.

Treatment of diabetes and diabetic complications with a ketogenic diet - 2013

Aggressive tumors typically demonstrate a high glycolytic rate, which results in resistance to radiation therapy and cancer progression via several molecular and physiologic mechanisms. Intriguingly, many of these mechanisms utilize the same molecular pathways that are altered through calorie and/or carbohydrate restriction.

Important mechanisms include:

- improved DNA repair in normal, but not tumor cells;
- inhibition of tumor cell repopulation;
- redistribution of normal cells into more radioresistant phases of the cell cycle;
- normalization of the tumor vasculature;
- increasing the intrinsic radioresistance of normal cells

through ketone bodies but decreasing that of tumor cells by targeting glycolysis.

Calorie restriction and ketogenic diets may act synergistically with radiation therapy for the treatment of cancer patients and provide some guidelines for implementing these dietary interventions into clinical practice.

Calories, carbohydrates, and cancer therapy with radiation: exploiting the five R's through dietary manipulation. - 2014

If cancer is primarily a disease of energy metabolism, then rational strategies for cancer management should be found in those therapies that specifically target tumor cell energy metabolism. As glucose is the major fuel for tumor energy metabolism through lactate fermentation, the restriction of glucose becomes a prime target for management.

It is well known that ketones can replace glucose as an energy metabolite and can protect the brain from severe hypoglycemia, hence, the shift in energy metabolism associated with a low carbohydrate, high-fat ketogenic diet administered in restricted amounts can protect normal cells from glycolytic inhibition and the brain from hypoglycemia.

When systemic glucose availability becomes limiting, most normal cells of the body will transition their energy metabolism to fats and ketone bodies. Most tumor cells are unable to use ketone bodies for energy due to abnormalities in mitochondria structure or function, ketone bodies can also be toxic to some cancer cells.

Nutritional ketosis induces metabolic stress on tumor tissue that is selectively vulnerable to glucose deprivation, hence, metabolic stress will be greater in tumor cells than in normal cells when the whole body is transitioned away from glucose and to ketone bodies for energy. The metabolic shift from glucose metabolism to ketone body metabolism creates an anti-angiogenic, anti-inflammatory and pro-apoptotic environment within the tumor mass.

Cancer as a metabolic disease: implications for novel therapeutics. - 2014

The only known treatment of glucose transporter 1 deficiency syndrome is a ketogenic diet, which provides the brain with an alternative fuel, however concerns still remain about its effects on body and bone composition.

In adults with GLUT-1 deficiency syndrome on a ketogenic diet for 5 years there were no appreciable changes in weight and body composition, and no evidence of potential adverse effects on bone health.

Long-term effects of a ketogenic diet on body composition and bone mineralization in GLUT-1 deficiency syndrome: a case series. - 2014

Low to Moderate General Carbohydrate Restriction

In prescriptions for weight loss, carbohydrates are usually restricted as far as possible, since they are known to be the principal source of surplus energy in the obese.

Subjects were put on diets of varying macronutrient levels, and differences of up to 400% in extra weight loss was noted the lower the carbohydrate intake was.

The Treatment of Obesity: A Comparison of the Effects of Diet and of Thyroid Extract. - 1932

The rate of weight loss has been shown to be proportional to the deficiency in calorie intake when the proportions of macronutrients are kept constant, however, the rate of weight loss varies greatly on diets of different composition.

When calorie intake was constant at 1,000 per day, it was most rapid with high-fat diets; it was less rapid with high-protein diets; and weight could be maintained for short periods on diets of chiefly carbohydrate.

At 2,000 calories per day, weight was maintained or increased in four out of five obese patients unless on the low-carb diet, and significant weight loss still occurred when calorie intake was raised to 2,600 per day, provided this intake was given mainly in the form of fat and protein.

Calorie intake in relation to body-weight changes in the obese. - 1956

5 subjects underwent a week of carbohydrate restriction which:

- lowered fasting insulin
- increased fasting glucagon
- reduced insulin/glucagon ratio
- reduced the insulin response to protein
- increased glucagon response to protein
- maintained the insulin/glucagon ratio when consuming protein

One week of restoration of carbohydrate to the diet:

- increased fasting insulin
- lowered fasting glucagon
- restored the insulin/glucagon ratio to previous levels
- further increased the insulin response to protein
- suppressed the glucagon response to protein
- caused the insulin/glucagon ratio to become very unbalanced

The Influence of the Antecedent Diet upon Glucagon and Insulin Secretion.

- 1971

On an 1,800 calorie diet with carbohydrates restricted to between 30-104g for 9 weeks, weight loss, fat loss, and percent weight loss as fat appeared to be inversely related to the level of carbohydrate.

Effect on body composition and other parameters in obese young men of carbohydrate level of reduction diet. - 1971

8 women were restricted to 80g of carbohydrate a day but protein and fat were allowed freely. Energy intake

was found to be ~30% lower on this diet than on the subject's habitual diet, but the nutrient content was not reduced.

During the 6 weeks of the dietary period, there was no change in triglycerides, cholesterol, or uric acid. The urinary excretion of nitrogen and creatinine were unchanged, indicating no significant loss of tissue protein.

The Absence of Undesirable Changes during Consumption of the Low Carbohydrate Diet. - 1974

During and after strenuous prolonged exercise, sedentary individuals develop high blood levels of ketones whereas exercise-trained animals and human subjects do not.

The trained animals had markedly lower blood ketone levels immediately and 60 min after a 90 min long bout of exercise than did the sedentary animals.

Exercise-induced increase in the capacity of rat skeletal muscle to oxidize ketones. - 1975

A test meal containing gelatin plus glucose resulted in much higher levels of insulin and increased insulin-glucagon ratio, lower glucagon levels, and slightly higher triglycerides than a meal of the same size of gelatin alone.

One week of very low carbohydrate ~2,800 calorie diet lowered insulin, the insulin-glucagon ratio, and triglycerides, plus increased glucagon.

Swapping back ~390g of carbohydrate significantly

increased insulin, the insulin-glucagon ratio, and triglycerides, and lowered glucagon within 2 days; even greater changes in hormones were observed on a 510g of carbohydrate.

Basal and postprotein insulin and glucagon levels during a high and low carbohydrate intake and their relationships to plasma triglycerides. - 1975

Electroencephalographic sleep changes were studied in subjects who were given a normal balanced diet or a high-carbohydrate/low-fat or low-carbohydrate/high-fat isocaloric diet.

Both high-carbohydrate/low-fat and low-carbohydrate/high-fat isocaloric diets, especially the former, were associated with significantly more rapid-eye-movement sleep than was the normal balanced diet.

Isocaloric diet changes and electroencephalographic sleep. - 1975

45 obese subjects were fed a high-carbohydrate, relatively low-fat, or a low-carbohydrate, relatively high-fat 1,000-calorie formula diet.

Weight reduction up to day 30 was significantly higher in the subjects on the carbohydrate-restricted diet. There were no significant differences between the water and electrolyte balances.

The mean total weight reduction achieved on the high-carbohydrate diet was ~9.8kg with a mean daily weight loss of ~298g, while the carbohydrate-restricted diet saw ~14kg and ~362g/day weight lost.

Comparative studies in obese subjects fed carbohydrate-restricted and

A high carbohydrate feeding can result in elevated levels of carbon dioxide waste due to increased usage of glucose as an energy source. In a normal ventilation situation this is typically incosequential.

In this case 3 patients needing ventilatory support were provided a high carbohydrate parenteral solution (intravenous feeding), hypercapnia (elevated blood CO2) ensued, followed by acute respiratory failure.

Respiratory failure precipitated by high carbohydrate loads. - 1981

10 diabetic patients were randomly assigned in crossover design a diet of either low fat high carb or moderate fat moderate carb each for 28 days.

The moderate diet resulted in lower glucose and reduced insulin requirements, lower triglycerides and VLDL-C, and higher HDL-C.

Comparison of a High-Carbohydrate Diet with a High-Monounsaturated-Fat Diet in Patients with Non-Insulin-Dependent Diabetes Mellitus. - 1988

8 men with mild diabetes were randomly put on either a low fat high carb or moderate fat and carb diet one after the other for 3 weeks.

The high-carbohydrate diet caused a significant increase in triglycerides and VLDL-cholesterol, and reduced HDL-cholesterol.

Women with gestational diabetes on either a high or moderate carb diet were studied.

In the lower-carbohydrate group there were significant reductions in postprandial glucose, fewer subjects required the addition of insulin for glucose control, the incidence of large for gestational age infants was significantly lower, and they had a lower rate of cesarean deliveries for cephalopelvic disproportion and macrosomia.

The effects of carbohydrate restriction in patients with diet-controlled gestational diabetes. - 1998

Subjects with type 2 diabetes were placed on a 25% carbohydrate diet for 8 weeks then switched to a 55% carbohydrate diet.

After the lower carb diet subjects showed significantly improved fasting glucose and hemoglobin A1c levels, but when switched to the high carbohydrate diet the hemoglobin A1c rose significantly.

Utility of a short-term 25% carbohydrate diet on improving glycemic control in type 2 diabetes mellitus. - 1998

20 women completed an 8-week trial that reduced their daily carbohydrate intake from ~232g to ~71g without

changes in protein or fat consumption. The diet promotes weight loss, and improvements in body composition, blood pressure, and blood lipids without compromising glucose tolerance in moderately overweight women.

Effects of a hypocaloric, low-carbohydrate diet on weight loss, blood lipids, blood pressure, glucose tolerance, and body composition in free-living overweight women. - 2002

Randomized trials are the preferable method to evaluate the effect of dietary fat on adiposity. In short-term trials, a modest reduction in body weight is typically seen in individuals randomized to diets with a lower percentage of calories from fat. However, compensatory mechanisms appear to operate, because in randomized trials lasting >or=1 year, fat consumption within the range of 18% to 40% of energy appears to have little if any effect on body fatness.

Moreover, within the United States, a substantial decline in the percentage of energy from fat during the last 2 decades has corresponded with a massive increase in the prevalence of obesity.

Diets high in fat do not appear to be the primary cause of the high prevalence of excess body fat in our society, and reductions in fat will not be a solution.

Dietary fat is not a major determinant of body fat. - 2002

24 women with BMI >26 were assigned to either a high carb/moderate protein or moderate carb/high protein diet of 1,700 calories, with ~50g coming from fat in each, therefore only modulating the protein and carbohydrate

loads.

The high carb diet followed the USDA Food Pyramid which emphasizes the use of breads, rice, cereals and pasta. The high protein diet substituted foods that emphasized animal proteins including red meats, milk, cheese and eggs, with a requirement for a minimum of seven beef meals each week.

After 10 weeks both groups lost similar amounts of bodyweight (~7-7.5kg), but the high protein group was partitioned to a significantly higher loss of fat vs lean than in the high carb group (~6.3kg vs ~3.8kg).

The high protein group had significant reductions in triglycerides and the ratio of TAG/HDL cholesterol.

Women in the high carb group had higher insulin responses to meals and postprandial hypoglycemia, whereas the high protein dieters reported greater satiety.

A reduced ratio of dietary carbohydrate to protein improves body composition and blood lipid profiles during weight loss in adult women. - 2003

8 men were randomized on a 5-week crossover between a normal high carb and a low carb diet.

The mean 24h integrated serum glucose at the end of the control diet was 198, at the end of the low carb diet it was 126. Glycohemoglobin dropped from ~9.8 to ~7.6, and was still decreasing at the end. Insulin was decreased, and glucagon was increased.

Effect of a high-protein, low-carbohydrate diet on blood glucose control in people with type 2 diabetes. - 2004

235 postmenopausal women with established coronary heart disease were studied for 3 years.

A greater saturated fat intake is associated with a smaller decline in mean minimal coronary diameter and less progression of coronary stenosis.

Carbohydrate intake was positively associated with atherosclerotic progression particularly when the glycemic index was high.

Polyunsaturated fat intake was positively associated with progression when replacing other fats but not when replacing carbohydrate or protein.

Dietary fats, carbohydrate, and progression of coronary atherosclerosis in postmenopausal women. - 2004

Different diets lead to different biochemical pathways that are not equivalent when correctly compared through the laws of thermodynamics. It is inappropriate to assume that the only thing that counts in terms of food consumption and energy balance is the intake of dietary calories and weight storage.

Diets high in fat do not appear to be the primary cause of obesity, and reductions in fat will not be the solution. The hormonal changes associated with a low-carbohydrate diet include a reduction in the circulating levels of insulin along with increased levels of glucagons, leading to activation of various pathways, favoring gluconeogenesis over glycolysis. There is evidence that hyperinsulinemia increases fat mass without a concomitant increase in energy intake.

It is increasingly clear that the idea that "a calorie is a calorie" is misleading. The calorie content may not be as predictive of fat loss as is reduced carbohydrate consumption. The ideal weight loss diet, if it even exists, remains to be determined, but a high-carbohydrate/low-protein diet may be unsatisfactory for many obese individuals.

Is a Calorie Really a Calorie? Metabolic Advantage of Low-Carbohydrate Diets. - 2004

A high intake of carbohydrates increases the risk of symptomatic gall stone disease in men. These results add to the concern that low fat high carbohydrate diets may not be an optimal dietary recommendation.

Dietary carbohydrates and glycaemic load and the incidence of symptomatic gall stone disease in men. - 2005

48 women with BMI >26 were assigned to either a high carb/moderate protein or moderate carb/high protein diet of 1,700 calories. These groups were then also split into either normal light activity or frequent walking and occasional resistance exercise, averaging ~3.5 hours exercise a week.

The high carb diet followed the USDA Food Pyramid which emphasizes restricting fat/cholesterol and the use of breads, rice, cereals and pasta. The high protein diet substituted meats, dairy, and eggs.

All groups lost significant weight during the 16 weeks, the lower carb groups moreso than the high carb groups (~9.3kg vs ~7.3kg).

The exercise treatment did not affect weight loss,

however those in the exercise groups lost more fat vs lean than the non-exercise groups.

Subjects in the high carb groups had larger reductions in total and LDL cholesterol, whereas subjects in the high protein groups had greater reductions in triglyceride and maintained higher concentrations of HDL cholesterol.

Dietary protein and exercise have additive effects on body composition during weight loss in adult women. - 2005

In a small group of obese patients with type 2 diabetes, a low-carbohydrate diet followed for 2 weeks resulted in spontaneous reduction in energy intake to a level appropriate to their height; weight loss that was completely accounted for by reduced caloric intake; much improved 24-hour blood glucose profiles, insulin sensitivity, and hemoglobin A1c; and decreased plasma triglyceride and cholesterol levels.

Effect of a low-carbohydrate diet on appetite, blood glucose levels, and insulin resistance in obese patients with type 2 diabetes. - 2005

Metabolic Syndrome (MetS) represents a constellation of markers that indicates a predisposition to diabetes, cardiovascular disease and other pathologic states.

Carbohydrate restriction is one of several strategies for reducing body mass but even in the absence of weight loss or in comparison with low fat alternatives, CHO restriction is effective at ameliorating high fasting glucose and insulin, high plasma triglycerides (TAG), low HDL and high blood pressure.

In addition, low fat, high CHO diets have long been known to raise TAG, lower HDL and, in the absence of weight loss, may worsen glycemic control.

Recent studies suggest that a subset of MetS, the ratio of TAG/HDL, is a good marker for insulin resistance and risk of CVD, and this indicator is reliably reduced by CHO restriction and exacerbated by high CHO intake.

Carbohydrate restriction improves the features of Metabolic Syndrome. Metabolic Syndrome may be defined by the response to carbohydrate restriction. - 2005

178 men with a BMI ~29 were put on either a normal high carb (59%), a reduced carb (39%), or moderate carb (26%) diet - with one of the moderate carb groups being assigned low saturated fat, the other high. All diets were restricted by ~1,000 calories, and weight loss over 3 weeks was ~5kg across the board.

After a further 4 weeks of weight stable energy intakes, the 26% carb diets both reduced trigs, apopB, total/HDL cholesterol ratio, and increased LDL sizes. The high sat fat further increased the mass of larger LDLs.

Separate effects of reduced carbohydrate intake and weight loss on atherogenic dyslipidemia. - 2006

Compared to weight loss on a low fat diet, a high saturated fat low carb diet with no weight loss resulted in better improvements in LDL peak size, TAG, HDL, and the ratios total cholesterol/HDL and apoB/ApoA-1.

Carbohydrate restriction alone is significantly better than

weight loss on a low fat diet for improving atherogenic dyslipidemia biomarkers.

Low carbohydrate diets improve atherogenic dyslipidemia even in the absence of weight loss. - 2006

Five trials including a total of 447 individuals assigned randomly to either low carb or low fat diets were meta-analysed.

After 6 months, individuals assigned to low-carbohydrate diets had lost more weight than those on low-fat diets, but after 12 months there was no significant difference.

Triglycerides were reduced and HDL cholesterol values increased on the low-carbohydrate diets, total cholesterol and LDL cholesterol values lowered in low-fat diets.

Effects of low-carbohydrate vs low-fat diets on weight loss and cardiovascular risk factors: A meta-analysis of randomized controlled trials. - 2006

102 patients with Type 2 diabetes were randomly allocated to a restricted carbohydrate or a reduced-portion, low-fat diet.

Weight loss was greater in the low-carbohydrate group (~3.5kg vs. ~0.9kg) and cholesterol:HDL ratio improved.

Short-term effects of severe dietary carbohydrate-restriction advice in Type 2 diabetes—a randomized controlled trial. - 2006

29 overweight men consumed an ad libitum low carb (13%) diet for 12 weeks.

Energy intake was spontaneously reduced by ~30%. Subjects lost ~7.5kg, and there were reductions in plasma Lp(a), LDL-C, CRP, and TNF-α.

Effects of a carbohydrate-restricted diet on emerging plasma markers for cardiovascular disease. - 2006

An obese patient with type 2 diabetes whose diet was changed from the recommended high-carbohydrate, low-fat type to a low-carbohydrate diet showed a significant reduction in bodyweight, improved glycemic control and a reversal of a 6 year long decline of renal function.

A low-carbohydrate diet may prevent end-stage renal failure in type 2 diabetes. A case report. - 2006

Moderately obese subjects consumed 2 different low carb diets as part of a weight loss regimen:

1) a diet high in foods of mammalian origin intended to contain more saturated fat, or

2) a diet high in poultry, fish, and shellfish, intended to contain more PUFA.

Both diets were associated with significant weight loss after 28 days. Despite high cholesterol and fat intakes, neither diet was associated with significant changes in plasma cholesterol or the plasma lipoprotein cholesterol profile. While plasma triglycerides were reduced in both groups, the effect was only statistically significant for the PFS diet.

The persistence of an epidemic of obesity, metabolic syndrome, and type 2 diabetes suggests that new nutritional strategies are needed if the epidemic is to be overcome.

Recent studies show that, under conditions of carbohydrate restriction, fuel sources shift from glucose and fatty acids to fatty acids and ketones, and that ad libitum–fed carbohydrate-restricted diets lead to appetite reduction, weight loss, improvement in hypertension, hyperlipidemia, glucose, triglycerides, HDL cholesterol, abdominal circumference, blood pressure, epilepsy and narcolepsy, and regulate surrogate markers of cardiovascular disease.

Low-carbohydrate nutrition and metabolism. - 2007

55 people of ~33 BMI were put on diets restricted by ~500 calories for 4 months, of either 1.6g/kg protein and <170g carbohydrate, or 0.8g/kg protein and >220g carbohydrate.

There was a trend for lower carb to lose more weight (~9.1% vs ~7.3%), and also favored reductions in triglyceride (~34% vs ~14%), and increases in HDL-C.

Insulin responses to the meal challenge were significantly improved in lower compared to higher carb at both 1 and 2 hours.

Moderate carbohydrate, moderate protein weight loss diet reduces

8 men with untreated type 2 diabetes were put on a moderate carbohydrate (30%) weight-maintenance diet for 5 weeks. Fasting glucose concentration decreased by 40%; 24h glucose area response decreased by 45%. Insulin did not change. Mean total glycohaemoglobin decreased by 1.7, and was still decreasing linearly at 5 weeks.

Effect of the LoBAG30 diet on blood glucose control in people with type 2 diabetes. - 2008

Dietary carbohydrate restriction in the treatment of diabetes is based on an underlying principle of controlling chronic hyperglycemia and therefore hyperinsulinemia. It has generally been opposed by health agencies because of concern that carbohydrate will be replaced by fat, particularly saturated fat.

Removing the barrier of concern about dietary fat makes carbohydrate restriction a reasonable, if not the preferred method for treating type 2 diabetes, considering the ability of low carbohydrate diets to improve glycemic control, hemoglobin A1C, and to reduce medication.

Carbohydrate restriction as the default treatment for type 2 diabetes and metabolic syndrome. - 2008

Subjects with type 2 diabetes on a low carbohydrate

diet after 6 months had lost ~11kg. In a follow-up after the intervention period at 22 months, mean bodyweight had increased by ~2.7kg, and at 44 months average weight has increased another ~1kg.

Of the 16 patients, 5 have retained or reduced bodyweight since the 22 month point and all but one have lower weight at 44 months than at start.

The initial mean HbA1c was ~8.0, after 6, 12 and 22 months, HbA1c was ~6.1, ~7.0, and ~6.9 respectively. After 44 months mean HbA1c is ~6.8.

Of the 23 patients who have used a low-carbohydrate diet and for whom we have long-term data, 2 have suffered a cardiovascular event while 4 of the 6 controls who never changed diet have suffered several cardiovascular events.

Low-carbohydrate diet in type 2 diabetes: stable improvement of bodyweight and glycemic control during 44 months follow-up. - 2008

10 recreationally active women, aged 25-40 years, followed an isoenergetic (30% fat) moderate-protein high-carb diet and a high-protein moderate-carb diet for a week each in a random counterbalanced design.

Body weight, body fat and respiratory exchange ratio were significantly reduced following the high-protein diet, but no differences were found in any of the strength performance parameters or the responses of heart rate, systolic and diastolic arterial pressure, blood lactate and blood glucose to exercise.

An isoenergetic high-protein, moderate-fat diet does not compromise strength and fatigue during resistance exercise in women. - 2008

In the early 20th century, before any medications were available for the treatment of diabetes mellitus, experts recommended dietary carbohydrate-restriction.

The dietary recommendation for diabetes in a prominent internal medicine textbook from 1923 was 75% fat, 17% protein, 6% alcohol and only 2% carbohydrate.

After the discovery of insulin and oral hypoglycemic medications, experts gradually changed the dietary recommendations to include more carbohydrate intake because most experts reasoned that the medications could be used to keep the glucose in control.

Has carbohydrate-restriction been forgotten as a treatment for diabetes mellitus? A perspective on the ACCORD study design. - 2008

Dietary carbohydrate is the major determinant of postprandial glucose levels, and several clinical studies have shown that low-carbohydrate diets improve glycemic control.

A diet lower in carbohydrate led to greater improvements in glycemic control, and more frequent medication reduction/elimination than a low glycemic index diet. Lifestyle modification using low carbohydrate interventions is effective for improving and reversing type 2 diabetes.

The effect of a low-carbohydrate, ketogenic diet versus a low-glycemic index diet on glycemic control in type 2 diabetes mellitus. - 2008

In a retrospective review of patients attending an outpatient metabolic management program 31 patients aged ~58 were prescribed a high fat low carb diet.

Body weight, serum leptin, insulin, fasting glucose, triglyceride, and free T(3) significantly decreased, Furthermore, the triglyceride/HDL ratio decreased from ~5.1 to ~2.6.

In the context of an outpatient medical clinic, a high-fat, adequate-protein, low-carbohydrate diet with nutritional supplementation led to improvements in serum factors related to the aging process.

Clinical Experience of a Diet Designed to Reduce Aging. - 2009

Subjects were put on a diet restricted by ~500 calories comprised of either 1.6g/kg of protein and <170g of carbohydrates, or 0.8g/kg of protein and >220g of carbs.

After 4 months the protein group had lost slightly more weight (~8.2kg vs ~7kg) and fat mass (~5.6kg vs ~4.6kg). At 12 months the rate of attrition was high, the lower carb group had more participants complete the study (64% vs 45%) with greater improvement in body composition, and weight loss was not significant (~10.4kg vs ~8.4kg).

The high carb diet reduced total and LDL cholesterol more at 4 months, but the effect did not remain at 12 months. Lower carb group had sustained favorable effects on trigs, HDL cholesterol, and TAG:HDL-C ratio compared with high carb at 4 and 12 months.

A moderate-protein diet produces sustained weight loss and long-term changes in body composition and blood lipids in obese adults. - 2009

This systematic review included all known RCTs of low-carb diets vs the low-fat/high-carb diet from 2000 to 2007. Factors including weight, cholesterol, blood pressure and glycemic control were evaluated, as these are important in weight loss and cardiovascular disease risk.

Evidence from this systematic review demonstrates that low carb diets are more effective at 6 months and are as effective, if not more, as low fat diets in reducing weight and cardiovascular disease risk up to 1 year.

Systematic review of randomized controlled trials of low-carbohydrate vs. low-fat/low-calorie diets in the management of obesity and its comorbidities. - 2009

200 overweight subjects were randomly assigned to a conventional low-fat (>55% carbs) or a moderate-carb diet (<40% carbs).

Energy intake decreased by ~400 calories within the first 6 months and slightly increased again within the second 6 months.

After 12 months the moderate carb group had lost ~5.8kg and the high carb group ~4.3kg.

Triglycerides, HDL-cholesterol, waist circumference and systolic blood pressure all improved more in the moderate carb group.

A randomized controlled trial on the efficacy of carbohydrate-reduced or fat-reduced diets in patients attending a telemedically guided weight loss program. - 2009

The prevalence of diabetes in the United Arab Emirates is among the highest world-wide.

The typical diet of Emirati people consists of fish, eggs, rice, bread, fruits, yogurt, vegetables, and wheat flour for desserts and meat wraps.

39 participants with metabolic syndrome followed a lowish-carb diet, they had no difficulty adapting to the CRD, which was followed by eliminating the rice and bread and reducing the yogurt and milk, and consuming only 1 fruit per day to bring carbohydrate down to ~25%.

After 6 weeks body weight decreased ~13% and plasma triglycerides dropped ~39%. Significant decreases in LDL cholesterol, blood pressure, glucose, insulin, and inflammatory markers, and increases in adiponectin also occurred.

After 6 weeks 19 were randomly switched to the AHA diet of 55% carbohydrate.

After 12 weeks, positive changes persisted for all participants, however, body weight and plasma TG and insulin were lower in the carb-restricted group than in the subjects who switched to the AHA diet.

Carbohydrate Restriction, as a First-Line Dietary Intervention, Effectively Reduces Biomarkers of Metabolic Syndrome in Emirati Adults. - 2009

69 participants (of 118, high attrition) completed a year of either very low carb or a standard diet, both of similar moderately restricted calories.

Both groups lost similar amounts of weight, the low carb group moderately moreso (~14kg vs ~11kg).

The low carb group had greater decreases in

triglycerides, increases in HDL cholesterol and LDL cholesterol.

Long-term effects of a very-low-carbohydrate weight loss diet compared with an isocaloric low-fat diet after 12 mo. - 2009

Exchanging carbohydrate for protein results in increased energy expenditure, fat oxidation, protein anabolism in men, and a stronger increased satiety in women.

Sex differences in energy homeostatis following a diet relatively high in protein exchanged with carbohydrate, assessed in a respiration chamber in humans. - 2009

Untrained overweight women were put on either a regular diet or low carb diet, and performed performed 60-100 min of varied resistance exercise twice weekly for 10 weeks.

Subjects on the low carb regime lost ~5.6kg of fat mass with no significant change in lean body mass, while the normal dieters gained ~1.6kg with no significant change in fat mass.

Resistance training in overweight women on a ketogenic diet conserved lean body mass while reducing body fat. - 2010

221 women participated in a 10-week exercise and weight loss program. The fitness program involved 30 minutes of resistance training 3 days per week. Subjects were prescribed low-fat diets with either high carb or low

carb.

Subjects in the low carb group experienced greater weight loss, fat loss, reductions in serum glucose, and decreases in serum leptin levels.

A carbohydrate-restricted diet during resistance training promotes more favorable changes in body composition and markers of health in obese women with and without insulin resistance. - 2011

That there exists an intimate connection between carbohydrates and cancer has been known since the seminal studies performed by different physiologists in the 1920s.

Hyperglycemia activates inflammatory cytokines that play an important role also for the progression of cancer, high plasma glucose concentrations elevate the levels of circulating insulin and free IGF1, two potent anti-apoptotic and growth factors for most cancer cells

Since 1885, when Ernst Freund described signs of hyperglycemia in 70 out of 70 cancer patients, it has been repeatedly reported that glucose tolerance and insulin sensitivity are diminished in cancer patients even before signs of cachexia (weight loss) become evident

It therefore seems reasonable to assume that dietary carbohydrates mainly fuel malignant cells, while muscle cells are more likely to benefit from an increased fat and protein intake.

Evidence has emerged from both animal and laboratory studies indicating that cancer patients could benefit further from a very low carbohydrate ketogenic diet.

Is There a Role for Carbohydrate Restriction in the Treatment and Prevention of Cancer? - 2011

Adiponectin is an adipose-derived protein with beneficial metabolic effects. 81 obese women in 2 cohorts (of 6 and 4 months) were randomized to a low-fat or a low-carbohydrate diet.

Weight loss in both cohorts was more significant in low carb groups (~9kg vs ~5kg). Adiponectin increased significantly more in the low carb group.

Adiponectin changes in relation to the macronutrient composition of a weight-loss diet. - 2011

Recent clinical research has studied weight responses to varying diet composition, but the contribution of changes in macronutrient intake and physical activity to rising population weight remains unknown. Findings from all analyses suggest that increases in carbohydrates are most strongly and positively associated with increases in obesity prevalence even when controlling for changes in total caloric intake and occupation-related physical activity.

If anything, increases in fat intake are associated with decreases in population weight.

Macronutrients and Obesity: Revisiting the Calories in, Calories out Framework - 2013

The aim of this study was to examine the effects of a non-calorie-restricted, low-carbohydrate diet in Japanese patients unable to adhere to a calorie-restricted diet.

A low-carbohydrate diet is effective in lowering the HbA1c and triglyceride levels in patients with type 2 diabetes who are unable to adhere to a low calorie diet.

A non-calorie-restricted low-carbohydrate diet is effective as an alternative therapy for patients with type 2 diabetes. - 2014

Two matched groups of ~52yo overweight type-2 diabetes patients without overt heart disease were studied in a parallel and partial cross-over design during a 3-week rehabilitation programme with either low carb or low fat followed by 2 weeks low carb.

Both diets induced similar and significant reductions of weight, HbA1c and cholesterol. Low carb considerably improved insulin resistance, fasting and postmeal triglycerides, blood pressure and diastolic cardiac function. None of these variables changed on low fat, but all of them improved significantly after subsequent low carb. Postprandial intact proinsulin was unchanged on low fat but decreased with subsequent low carb.

Low-carbohydrate/high-protein diet improves diastolic cardiac function and the metabolic syndrome in overweight-obese patients with type 2 diabetes.
- 2014

30 women with PCOS consumed a moderate carb and fat diet a standard high carb low fat diet for 8 weeks in a crossover design.

The reduced carb diet induced a decrease in subcutaneous-abdominal, intra-abdominal, and thighintermuscular fat, and the standard diet induced a decrease in total lean mass.

Effects of a eucaloric reduced-carbohydrate diet on body composition and fat distribution in women with PCOS. - 2014

In women with a primary breast cancer tumor that was positive for the insulin-like growth factor 1 receptor, an association was found between both tumor growth and cancer recurrence on a restricted carbohydrate diet.

Risk of Breast Cancer Recurrence Associated with Carbohydrate Intake and Tissue Expression of IGF-1 Receptor. - 2014

Animal Studies

During and after strenuous prolonged exercise, sedentary individuals develop high blood levels of ketones whereas exercise-trained animals and human subjects do not.

The trained animals had markedly lower blood ketone levels immediately and 60 min after a 90 min long bout of exercise than did the sedentary animals.

Exercise-induced increase in the capacity of rat skeletal muscle to oxidize ketones. - 1975

Racing sled dogs trained to maximal fitness were put on a zero, lowish, or moderate carbohydrate diet.

No adverse effects were observed in dogs on zero carb, and maintained higher concentrations of albumin, calcium, magnesium, and free fatty acids during the racing season. They also exhibited the greatest increases in red cell count, hemoglobin concentration, and packed cell volume during training.

High values of red cells were not sustained through the racing season in dogs fed the higher carb diet.

The carbohydrate-free, high-fat diet appeared to confer advantages for prolonged strenuous running.

Hematological and metabolic responses to training in racing sled dogs fed diets containing medium, low, or zero carbohydrate. - 1977

Cancer cell growth in culture was inhibited by ketone bodies and this effect was reversible, non-toxic, and proportional to the concentration of ketone bodies. D-beta-hydroxybutyrate was not metabolised by the cells.

Dietary-induced ketosis reduced the number of melanoma deposits in the lungs of mice by two-thirds.

THE INHIBITION OF MALIGNANT CELL GROWTH BY KETONE BODIES. - 1979

In situations where mice are severely deprived of oxygen, ketogenic subjects cope and survive much better than normal mice.

Hypoxia induced preferential ketone utilization by rat brain slices. - 1984

Rats were randomly put on either a LCHF diet or a normal diet, after a week the LCHF rats endurance to exhaustion was ~8% longer, and the gap increased to ~33% after five weeks.

Adaptations to LCHF included lower glycogen in both liver and muscles, and decreased glycogen breakdown during exercise, demonstrating high glycogen loads are unnecessary for endurance.

There was also decreased lactate production and increased fatty acid metabolism enzyme activity.

Adaptations to a high-fat diet that increase exercise endurance in male rats. - 1984

Recent evidence has shown that when the organism adapts to a high fat diet endurance is not hindered.

Fat-adapted rats ran as long as carbohydrate-fed animals in spite of lower pre-exercise glycogen levels.

Glycogen repletion and exercise endurance in rats adapted to a high fat diet - 1990

Rats adapted to a prolonged high fat diet increase maximal O2 uptake and submaximal running endurance.

Additive effects of training and high-fat diet on energy metabolism during exercise - 1991

Parkinson's disease is a neurodegenerative disorder of the central nervous system, resulting in various motor system and psychological problems.

It is demonstrated that an infusion into mice of the ketone body DβHB, a crucial alternative source of glucose for brain energy, confers protection against the structural and functional deleterious effects of the parkinsonian toxin MPTP.

DβHB levels may be a straightforward neuroprotective strategy for the treatment of neurodegenerative diseases.

D-β-Hydroxybutyrate rescues mitochondrial respiration and mitigates features of Parkinson disease. - 2003

Ketones displace glucose as the predominating fuel for the brain, decreasing the need for glucose synthesis and accordingly spares its precursor, muscle-derived amino acids.

In a rats heart it increased contractility and decreased oxygen consumption. It has also protected neuronal cells in tissue culture against exposure to toxins associated with Alzheimer's or Parkinson's.

In a rodent model it decreased the death of lung cells induced by hemorrhagic shock. Also, mice exposed to oxygen deprivation survived longer.

Ketoacids? Good medicine? - 2003

Despite having similar mean bodyweight, rats given high-GI food had more body fat and less lean body mass than those given low-GI food. The high-GI group also had greater increases over time in blood glucose and plasma insulin after oral glucose, lower plasma adiponectin concentrations, higher triglycerides, and severe disruption of islet-cell architecture.

Mice on the high-GI diet had almost twice the body fat of those on the low-GI diet after 9 weeks.

Effects of dietary glycaemic index on adiposity, glucose homoeostasis, and plasma lipids in animals. - 2004

In animal models of depression, test scores of rats on the ketogenic diet were compared with those of rats on a control diet. Rats on the ketogenic diet spent less time immobile, suggesting that like rats treated with antidepressants, are less likely to exhibit "behavioral despair".

The antidepressant properties of the ketogenic diet. - 2004

Normal and diabetic rats were fed either a regular or low-carbohydrate diet for 30 or 90 days. All diabetic control animals developed cataracts, no treated diabetic animals developed cataracts. There were no deleterious effects on retinal antioxidant defenses with either a 30-d or chronic low-carbohydrate diet.

Effects of low-carbohydrate diet and Pycnogenol treatment on retinal antioxidant enzymes in normal and diabetic rats. - 2006

The pattern of protection of the ketogenic diet in animal models of seizures is distinct from that of other anticonvulsants, suggesting that it has a unique mechanism of action. During consumption of the ketogenic diet, marked alterations in brain energy metabolism occur, with ketone bodies partly replacing glucose as fuel.

In addition to acute seizure protection, the ketogenic diet has neuroprotective properties in diverse models of neurodegenerative disease.

The Neuropharmacology of the Ketogenic Diet. - 2007

Many current therapies for malignant brain tumors fail to provide long-term management because they ineffectively target tumor cells while negatively impacting the health and vitality of normal brain cells. In contrast to brain tumor cells, which lack metabolic flexibility and are largely dependent on glucose for growth and survival, normal brain cells can metabolize both glucose and ketone bodies for energy.

Adult mice were implanted with malignant brain tumors and put on an either unrestricted or restricted ketogenic diet, the effects on tumor growth, vascularity, and survival were compared with that of an unrestricted high carbohydrate standard diet.

The restricted keto diet reduced glucose levels while elevating ketone body levels, significantly decreased the growth of the tumors, and significantly enhanced health and survival compared to that of the control groups receiving the standard low fat/high carbohydrate diet.

Gene expression was lower in the tumors than in the contralateral normal brain suggesting that these brain tumors have reduced ability to metabolize ketone bodies for energy.

The calorically restricted ketogenic diet, an effective alternative therapy for malignant brain cancer. - 2007

Dietary protocols that increase serum levels of ketones, such as calorie restriction and the ketogenic diet, offer robust protection against a multitude of acute and chronic neurological diseases. The underlying mechanisms, however, remain unclear.

It is demonstrated that ketones reduce glutamate-induced free radical formation and enhancing mitochondrial respiration in neocortical neurons. This mechanism may, in part, contribute to the neuroprotective activity of ketones by restoring normal bioenergetic function in the face of oxidative stress.

KETONES INHIBIT MITOCHONDRIAL PRODUCTION OF REACTIVE OXYGEN SPECIES PRODUCTION FOLLOWING GLUTAMATE EXCITOTOXICITY BY INCREASING NADH OXIDATION. - 2007

Mice were fed one of four diets: a ketogenic diet; an obesegenic diet high in fat and carbohydrate; a calorie restricted diet; and a control diet.

The keto, obesegenic, and control diets were all the same amount of calories.

Mice on keto and calorie restricted both dropped to ~85% of initial weight.

Keto mice formed a unique gene expression which promoted fatty acid oxidation and reduction in fat synthesis.

Mice made obese on the high fat/carb diet were then put on keto and lost all excess weight, improved glucose tolerace, and spontaneously increased energy expenditure.

A high-fat, ketogenic diet induces a unique metabolic state in mice. - 2007

Rats were fed a normal, high carbohydrate, or ketogenic diet for 19 weeks.

Electron microscopes demonstrate a decrease in the number of mitochondria when fed a high carbohydrate diet and an increase in those fed a ketogenic diet.

Keto subjects had a remarkable tolerance to restriction of blood supply to the heart, and a faster recovery of cardiac function following blood-restricted damage.

Low carbohydrate ketogenic diet enhances cardiac tolerance to global ischaemia. - 2007

Despite consuming more calories, zero carbohydrate ketogenic fed mice had significantly reduced tumor growth and prolonged survival relative to Western mice, and was associated with favorable changes in serum insulin and insulin-like growth hormones relative to low-fat or Western diet.

Carbohydrate restriction, prostate cancer growth, and the insulin-like growth factor axis. - 2008

Ketone bodies demonstrate a scavenging capacity for diverse reactive oxygen species, reducing cell death and reactive oxygen species production, prevention of neuronal ATP decline, and prevention of the hypoglycemia-induced increase in lipid peroxidation in the rat hippocampus.

Antioxidant capacity contributes to protection of ketone bodies against oxidative damage induced during hypoglycemic conditions. - 2008

Ketone bodies have been shown to be favorable alternative metabolic substrates and are protective under neuropathologies.

At the same time, cytochrome c release has been reported following traumatic brain injury and precipitates apoptosis (cell death) via the mitochondrial pathway.

Animals with traumatic brain injury were fed either normal or ketogenic diet.

The results show that brain edema, cytochrome c release, and cellular apoptosis were induced after traumatic brain injury and that a ketogenic diet reduced these changes dramatically.

Ketogenic diet reduces cytochrome c release and cellular apoptosis following traumatic brain injury in juvenile rats - 2009

Adult rats were divided into 3 groups: normal diet, keto, and high-carbohydrate diet. Diabetes was induced by injection.

The results showed that a ketogenic diet was effective in bringing blood glucose level close to normal. Food and water intake and urine output were increased in all groups except the keto group. The body weight was significantly reduced in all diabetic animals except in the keto group.

This study indicates that a ketogenic diet has a significant beneficial effect in ameliorating the diabetic state and helping to stabilize hyperglycemia.

Therapeutic role of low-carbohydrate ketogenic diet in diabetes. - 2009

To test the effects of a ketone-based metabolism on pain and inflammation directly, rats were fed a control diet or ketogenic diet ad libitum for 3–4 weeks. They were then subject to hindpaw thermal nociception (burning their feet) as a pain measure.

Independent of age, maintenance on a ketogenic diet reduced the peripheral inflammatory response significantly as measured by paw swelling and plasma extravasation. The ketogenic diet also induced significant thermal hypoalgesia independent of age, shown by increased hindpaw withdrawal latency in the hotplate nociception test.

Reduced Pain and Inflammation in Juvenile and Adult Rats Fed a Ketogenic Diet. - 2009

Aging is associated with increased susceptibility to hypoxic/ischemic insult and declines in behavioral function which may be due to attenuated adaptive/defense responses.

In aged rats, the ketogenic diet improved cognitive performance under normoxic and hypoxic conditions.

Diet-induced ketosis improves cognitive performance in aged rats. - 2010

The main clinical symptom of Parkinson's Disease is motor dysfunction derived from the loss of dopaminergic neurons in the substantia nigra and dopamine content in the striatum subsequently. It is well known that treatments with 1-methyl-4-phenyl-1,2,3,6-tetrahydropyridine (MPTP) in mice produce motor dysfunction, biochemical, and neurochemical changes remarkably similar to idiopathic Parkinson's patients.

Pre-treatment with a ketogenic diet alleviated the motor dysfunction induced by MPTP, the decrease of compromised neurons induced by MPTP was inhibited, and the activation of microglia was inhibited.

Neuroprotective and Anti-inflammatory Activities of Ketogenic Diet on MPTP-induced Neurotoxicity. - 2010

Mitochondrial dysfunction is a major cause of neurodegenerative and neuromuscular diseases of adult age and of multisystem disorders of childhood.

Mice which are a disease model for progressive late-onset mitochondrial myopathy were put on a ketogenic diet, the effects being a decrease in the amount of cytochrome c oxidase negative muscle fibers, a key feature in mitochondrial RC deficiencies, and prevented completely the formation of the mitochondrial ultrastructural abnormalities in the muscle.

Furthermore, most of the metabolic and lipidomic changes were cured by the diet. The diet did not, however, significantly affect the mtDNA quality or quantity, but rather induced mitochondrial biogenesis and restored liver lipid levels.

Ketogenic diet slows down mitochondrial myopathy progression in mice. - 2010

Rats which were fasted for 48 hours or following a ketogenic diet increased their ketone and glucose uptake more than 2-fold.

This approach may be particularly interesting in neurodegenerative pathologies such as Alzheimer's disease where brain energy supply appears to decline critically.

Mild experimental ketosis increases brain uptake of 11C-acetoacetate and 18F-fluorodeoxyglucose: a dual-tracer PET imaging study in rats. - 2011

In mouse models diabetic kidney disease was allowed to develop, then half the mice were switched to a ketogenic diet.

After 8 weeks it was completely reversed.

Reversal of Diabetic Nephropathy by a Ketogenic Diet. - 2011

As primarily a metabolic disease, malignant brain cancer can be managed through changes in metabolic environment. In contrast to normal neurons and glia, which readily transition to ketone bodies for energy under reduced glucose, malignant brain tumors are strongly dependent on glucose for energy.

This approach to brain cancer management is supported from recent studies in mice and humans treated with calorie restriction and the ketogenic diet.

Metabolic management of brain cancer. - 2011

Huntington's disease is a progressive neurodegenerative disease characterized by neurological, behavioral and metabolic dysfunction, and ketogenic diets have been shown to increase energy molecules and mitochondrial function.

Transgenic Huntington's mice were fed a ketogenic diet ad libitum. There were no usual Huntington's negative effects on any behavioral parameter tested and no significant change in lifespan. Progressive weight loss is a hallmark feature of Huntington's disease, yet the ketogenic diet delayed the reduction in body weight of the transgenic mice.

A ketogenic diet delays weight loss and does not impair working memory or motor function in the R6/2 1J mouse model of Huntington's disease. - 2011

Since cancer cells depend on glucose more than normal cells, the effects of low carbohydrate diets were compared to a Western diet on the growth rate of tumors in mice induced with cancer.

Tumors appeared in nearly 50% of mice on a Western diet within a year, whereas no tumors were detected in mice on the low carbohydrate diet.

Only 1 mouse on the Western diet achieved a normal life span, due to cancer-associated deaths. More than 50% of the mice on the low carbohydrate diet reached or exceeded the normal lifespan.

A Low Carbohydrate, High Protein Diet Slows Tumor Growth and Prevents Cancer Initiation. - 2011

Diet potently modulates the toxic effects of an acute lethal dose of the (chemical warfare) nerve agent soman.

In repeated doses of soman administration, rats fed the glucose-enriched diet showed pronounced intoxication during week 1, resulting in imperfect survival, weight loss, and deteriorated performance relative to all other groups. All rats fed the glucose-enriched diet died by the end of week 2.

Only 10% of animals fed the standard diet died by the end of week 2.

Survival in the standard and choline diet groups approximated 50% by week 3, whereas survival equaled 90% in the ketogenic diet group.

Diet composition modifies the toxicity of repeated soman exposure in rats.
- 2011

Rats were fed ad libitum for 8 weeks on either a normal diet, a high carb diet, or a ketogenic diet, then injected with streptozotocin - a chemical which is toxic to insulin-producing beta cells in the pancreas, thus inducing diabetes.

Blood glucose, food intake, water intake, urine output, and weight gain were significantly increased in all but the ketogenic rats.

A substantial decrease in the number of beta cells was noticed in all injected rats except for the ketogenic subjects.

Low carbohydrate ketogenic diet prevents the induction of diabetes using streptozotocin in rats. - 2011

Amyotrophic lateral sclerosis (AKA Lou Gehrig's disease and the disorder affecting Stephen Hawking) is a neurodegenerative disorder of motor neurons causing progressive muscle weakness, paralysis, and finally death.

When fed a ketogenic diet, the ALS mouse shows a significant increase in serum ketones as well as a significantly slower progression of weakness and lower mortality rate.

Treatment with MCT to promote ketone body generation attenuated progression of weakness and protected spinal cord motor neuron loss, significantly improving their performance even though there was no significant benefit regarding the survival of the ALS transgenic animals.

Caprylic triglyceride as a novel therapeutic approach to effectively improve the performance and attenuate the symptoms due to the motor neuron loss in ALS disease. - 2012

Following tumor implantation mice were maintained on standard diet or a ketogenic formula.

Keto diet plus radiation treatment were more than additive, and in 9 of 11 irradiated animals maintained on keto the tumor cells diminished below the level of detection.

They were switched to standard diet 101 days after implantation and no signs of tumor recurrence were seen for over 200 days.

The Ketogenic Diet Is an Effective Adjuvant to Radiation Therapy for the Treatment of Malignant Glioma. - 2012

2 year old rats were fed a ketogenic diet for 2 weeks, cerebral metabolic rates of ketones and glucose increased

significantly.

The ketogenic diet increases brain glucose and ketone uptake in aged rats:
a dual tracer PET and volumetric MRI study. - 2012

Treatment of cells in mice with ketone bodies conferred substantial protection against oxidative stress.

Suppression of oxidative stress by β-hydroxybutyrate, an endogenous
histone deacetylase inhibitor. - 2013

Central nervous system oxygen toxicity seizures occur with little or no warning, and no effective mitigation strategy has been identified.

Rats were administered a single oral dose of ketone esters to increase ketone body production, then placed into a hyperbaric chamber and pressurized to 5 atmospheres.

Latency to seizure was increased ~574%, the control subjects suffering siezures within ~11 minutes, the ketogenic rats taking almost an hour to capitulate such a fate.

Therapeutic ketosis with ketone ester delays central nervous system
oxygen toxicity seizures in rats. - 2013

Ketogenic diets are high in fat and low in carbohydrates which forces cells to rely on lipid oxidation and mitochondrial respiration rather than glycolysis for energy metabolism.

Mice with transplanted lung cancer were fed a ketogenic diet, combined with radiation resulted in slower tumor growth relative to radiation alone.

These results show that a ketogenic diet enhances radio-chemo-therapy responses in lung cancer xenografts by a mechanism that may involve increased oxidative stress.

Ketogenic Diets Enhance Oxidative Stress and Radio-Chemo-Therapy Responses in Lung Cancer Xenografts. - 2013

In young adult rats fed 3 weeks of either standard or ketogenic diets, cerebral metabolic rates of glucose significantly decreased in the cerebral cortex and cerebellum with increased plasma ketone bodies in the ketotic rats compared with standard diet group.

Ketosis proportionately spares glucose utilization in brain. - 2013

Cancer metabolism relies on glucose which can be exploited by lowering availability to the tumor. The ketogenic diet decreases blood glucose and has been shown to slow cancer progression. Hyperbaric oxygen therapy saturates tumors with oxygen, reversing cancer promoting effects.

Ketogenic diet alone significantly decreased blood glucose, slowed tumor growth, and increased mean survival time by ~56% in mice with systemic metastatic cancer. While hyperbaric therapy alone did not influence cancer progression, combining keto with hyperbaric therapy elicited a significant decrease in blood glucose, tumor growth rate, and ~78% increase in mean survival time compared to controls.

The Ketogenic Diet and Hyperbaric Oxygen Therapy Prolong Survival in Mice with Systemic Metastatic Cancer. - 2013

Rats fed a ketogenic diet for an extended period experienced decreased sensitivity to heat stimulated pain (thermal hypoalgesia), but it did not manifest until 10 days of keto, thus, ketosis and decreased glucose alone are not sufficient for hypoalgesia.

After just one day of returning to normal chow any pain sensitivity benefits were lost.

Ketogenic diets and thermal pain: dissociation of hypoalgesia, elevated ketones, and lowered glucose in rats. - 2013

Autism spectrum disorders share 3 core symptoms: impaired sociability, repetitive behaviors and communication deficits.

Juvenile mice with behavioural analogies to autism were fed a ketogenic diet for 3 weeks and tested, they showed increased sociability, decreased self-directed repetitive behavior, and improved social communication of a food preference.

Ketogenic diet improves core symptoms of autism in BTBR mice. - 2013

4 hours following spinal cord injury rats were fed either a standard carbohydrate based diet or a ketogenic diet.

The functional recovery was evaluated for 14 weeks, ketogenic diet treatment resulted in increased usage and range of motion of the affected forepaw. Furthermore, keto improved pellet retrieval with recovery of wrist and digit movements. Importantly, after returning to a standard diet after 12 weeks of keto treatment, the improved forelimb function remained stable.

The spinal cords of keto treated animals displayed smaller lesion areas and more grey matter sparing. Post-injury ketogenic diet effectively promotes functional recovery and is neuroprotective after spinal cord injury.

Ketogenic Diet Improves Forelimb Motor Function after Spinal Cord Injury
in Rodents. - 2013

Cancer cells express an abnormal metabolism characterized by increased glucose consumption owing to genetic mutations and mitochondrial dysfunction.

Previous studies indicate that unlike healthy tissues, cancer cells are unable to effectively use ketone bodies for energy.

Dietary ketone supplementation prolonged survival in mice with systemic metastatic cancer.

Ketone supplementation decreases tumor cell viability and prolongs
survival of mice with metastatic cancer - 2014

Heart Health, Metabolic Disorders, Blood Lipids, Cholesterol

11 subjects were prescribed a diet of 300-600ml of milk and as much meat, fish, eggs, cheese, butter, margarine, cream and leafy vegetables as they wished. The amount of carbohydrate in other food was limited to not more than 50g.

The low carbohydrate diet presents no health hazard, either generally or in regard to its nutritional value. The nutrient content is appreciably higher than could be achieved by a diet in which the same caloric reduction was effected by a general restriction in all foods.

Nutrient Intake of Subjects on Low Carbohydrate Diet Used in Treatment of Obesity. - 1970

Obese subjects were treated with a high fat low carbohydrate diet resulting in an average daily weight reduction of 0.3kg, the cholesterol and triglyceride concentrations in the serum, which had been raised at the beginning of the experiment, invariably showed a tendency towards normalization under this dietary program.

Response of body weight to a low carbohydrate, high fat diet in normal and obese subjects. - 1973

8 women were restricted to 80g of carbohydrate a day

but protein and fat were allowed freely.

During the 6 weeks of the dietary period, there was no change in the plasma concentration of triglyceride, cholesterol or uric acid.

The Absence of Undesirable Changes during Consumption of the Low Carbohydrate Diet. - 1974

One week of a 12 g/day carbohydrate, 2,870-calorie diet lowered triglycerides.

A 390 g/day carbohydrate, 2,784-calorie intake significantly increased triglycerides within 2 days.

Basal and postprotein insulin and glucagon levels during a high and low carbohydrate intake and their relationships to plasma triglycerides. - 1975

Two isocaloric reducing diets (10cal/kg bodyweight) were studied, one high in fat and low in carbohydrate content, the other high in carbohydrate and low in fat.

Fasting serum triglyceride and cholesterol levels declined to a greater extent following the high fat regimen. These changes reflected decrements in VLDL alone.

Effect of diet composition on metabolic adaptations to hypocaloric nutrition: comparison of high carbohydrate and high fat isocaloric diets. - 1977

To study the metabolic effects of ketosis without weight loss, nine lean men were fed a balanced diet for one week followed by four weeks of a ketogenic diet.

Serum cholesterol levels rose, while triglycerides fell, with no measurable impairment of hepatic, renal, cardiac, or hematopoietic function

.

The human metabolic response to chronic ketosis without caloric restriction: physical and biochemical adaptation. - 1983

For seven days before each study, distance runners consumed a diet containing 15% protein, 32% fat, and 53% carbohydrate.

During 14-day experimental periods, they consumed 69% of their calories as either carbohydrate or fat.

In the high-carbohydrate diet HDL cholesterol decreased, total and LDL cholesterol initially decreased but subsequently exceeded pre-diet values while triglyceride concentrations increased significantly.

The high-fat diet provided 111g of saturated fat per day but had little effect on total and LDL cholesterol, whereas triglycerides decreased.

The effects of high-carbohydrate and high-fat diets on the serum lipid and lipoprotein concentrations of endurance athletes. - 1984

Patients with diabetes were put on diets in a random crossover design of 15 days each, one low fat high carb resembling recommendations made by the American Diabetes Association, the other moderate fat and carbohydrate.

On the ADA diet fasting and postprandial triglyceride

levels were increased, HDL-C was reduced, and the HDL/LDL cholesterol ratio fell.

Deleterious metabolic effects of high-carbohydrate, sucrose-containing diets in patients with non-insulin-dependent diabetes mellitus. - 1987

7 patients with elevated cholesterol followed a diet in which most of the calories came from beef fat, the diets contained no sucrose, milk, or grains.

Triglyceride levels decreased from ~113 to ~74, cholesterol levels fell from ~263 to ~189.

6 of the patients started with a HDL percentage of ~21%, this rose to ~32%.

Reducing the serum cholesterol level with a diet high in animal fat. - 1988

10 diabetic patients were randomly assigned in crossover design a diet of either low fat high carb or moderate fat moderate carb each for 28 days.

The diet with more fat and less carbs resulted in lower triglycerides and VLDL-C, and higher HDL-C.

Comparison of a High-Carbohydrate Diet with a High-Monounsaturated-Fat Diet in Patients with Non-Insulin-Dependent Diabetes Mellitus. - 1988

Subjects were placed on diets of either low fat high carb or moderate fat and carb, consumed in random order for 6 weeks in a crossover design.

On the higher carb diet total and VLDL triglycerides increased significantly after 1 week, and the magnitude of carbohydrate-induced hypertriglyceridemia persisted unchanged throughout the 6 week study period.

Persistence of Hypertriglyceridemic Effect of Low-Fat High-Carbohydrate Diets in NIDDM Patients. - 1989

Serum lipoproteins, body composition, and adipose cholesterol contents of 6 obese women were studied during and after major weight loss by very-low-calorie diets.

Cholesterol fell significantly during the first 2 months, after which it rose above baseline as weight loss continued. With weight maintenance, cholesterol fell again.

It was concluded major weight loss was associated with a late rise in serum cholesterol, possibly from mobilization of adipose cholesterol stores, which resolved when weight loss ceased.

The transient hypercholesterolemia of major weight loss. - 1991

8 men with mild diabetes were randomly put on either a low fat high carb or moderate fat and carb diet one after the other for 3 weeks.

The high-carbohydrate diet caused a significant increase in triglycerides and VLDL-cholesterol, and reduced HDL-cholesterol.

Comparison of Effects of High and Low Carbohydrate Diets on Plasma Lipoproteins and Insulin Sensitivity in Patients With Mild NIDDM. - 1992

42 diabetic patients were put on a low fat high carb or moderate fat and carb diet for 6 weeks one after the other.

The high carb diet increased fasting and daylong triglycerides, as well as VLDL-cholesterol.

EFfects of varying carbohydrate content of diet in patients with non—insulin-dependent diabetes mellitus. - 1994

In a study of subjects with varying levels of cholesterol, swapping out carbohydrates for protein resulted in:

- significantly reduced LDL-C in subjects with normal and moderately high cholesterol
- significantly increased HDL-C and reduced ratio of total:HDL-C in those with moderate and familial hypercholesterolemia
- significantly reduced triglycerides in all groups

Potential role of raising dietary protein intake for reducing risk of atherosclerosis. - 1995

The commonly-held belief that the best diet for prevention of coronary heart disease is a low saturated fat, low cholesterol diet is not supported by the available evidence from clinical trials. In primary prevention, such diets do not reduce the risk of myocardial infarction or coronary or all-cause mortality.

Similarly, diets focused exclusively on reduction of saturated fats and cholesterol are relatively ineffective for secondary prevention and should be abandoned.

The low fat/low cholesterol diet is ineffective. - 1997

Positive correlations between intakes of fat and cardiovascular mortality found in earlier studies are absent or negative in larger, more recent studies.

Among 21 cohort studies of CHD including 28 cohorts, CHD patients had eaten significantly more SFA in 3 cohorts and significantly less in one cohort than had CHD-free individuals; in 22 cohorts no significant difference was noted. In 3 cohorts, CHD patients had eaten significantly more PUFA, in 24 cohorts no significant difference was noted.

In 3 of 4 cohort studies of atherosclerosis, the vascular changes were unassociated with SFA or PUFA; in one study they were inversely related to total fat. No significant differences in fat intake were noted in 6 case-control studies of CVD patients and CVD-free controls; and neither total or CHD mortality were lowered in a meta-analysis of nine controlled, randomized dietary trials with substantial reductions of dietary fats, in 6 trials combined with addition of PUFA.

The harmful effect of dietary SFA and the protective effect of dietary PUFA on atherosclerosis and CVD are not demonstrated conclusively.

The questionable role of saturated and polyunsaturated fatty acids in cardiovascular disease. - 1998

20 healthy volunteers consumed a moderate fat diet for 1 month, then for a 2nd month half of the subjects changed to a low-fat diet.

There was a decline in HDL-cholesterol after the low-fat diet and a small increase in the moderate-fat diet, with no significant changes in total cholesterol, LDL-C or triglyceride.

Triglycerides were measured after subjects ingested a single high fat meal, then were put on a ketogenic diet for 6 weeks and tested again.

Response to the meal after keto was decreased by half, demonstrating a profound improvement in metabolizing dietary fat.

This experiment has been successfully repeated on normal and overweight men and women.

Fasting lipoprotein and postprandial triglyceride responses to a low-carbohydrate diet supplemented with n-3 fatty acids. - 2000

19 non-obese males with elevated triglycerides received 2 consecutive diets for 3 weeks each: first a moderate-fat lower-carb diet with a focus on unsaturated fat, and then a low-fat higher-carb diet.

The higher-fat diet significantly DECREASED:

- triglycerides
- total cholesterol
- VLDL cholesterol
- LDL cholesterol
- total apoC-III
- apoC-III in apoB containing lipoproteins and in HDL
- apoE in serum and apoB-containing lipoproteins
- LpA-I
- insulin
- leptin

The higher-fat diet significantly INCREASED:

- HDL cholesterol
- LDL size
- lipoprotein lipase
- hepatic lipase
- and lecithin: cholesterol acyltransferase

The low-fat diet INCREASED:

- triglycerides
- VLDL cholesterol
- apoC-III
- apoC-III LpB
- apoC-III nonLpB
- apoE
- nonHDL-E

The low-fat diet DECREASED:

- HDL cholesterol
- LPL
- LCAT

Treatment of hypertriglyceridemia by two diets rich either in unsaturated fatty acids or in carbohydrates: effects on lipoprotein subclasses, lipolytic enzymes, lipid transfer proteins, insulin and leptin. - 2000

24 subjects completed a 12-week high monounsaturated fat, very low carbohydrate programme.

No adverse effects were recorded in any test. Subjects benefited by significant weight loss and a reduction in total cholesterol and triglycerides. HDL-C was unaffected.

Metabolic and Anthropometric changes in obese subjects from an unrestricted calorie, high monounsaturated fat, very low carbohydrate diet.
- 2000

For over 25 years eggs have been the icon for the fat, cholesterol and caloric excesses, and the message to limit eggs to lower heart disease risk has been widely circulated.

Cholesterol feeding studies demonstrate that dietary cholesterol increases both LDL and HDL cholesterol with little change in the LDL:HDL ratio, which would be predicted to have little effect on heart disease risk.

The impact of egg limitations on coronary heart disease risk: do the numbers add up? - 2000

An increase of up to 300% of dietary cholesterol intake had little effect on total or LDL cholesterol concentrations in healthy, postmenopausal women, irrespective of whether they were insulin-resistant or insulin-sensitive.

Insulin resistance, dietary cholesterol, and cholesterol concentration in postmenopausal women. - 2001

12 men switched from their habitual diet to a ketogenic diet and 8 control subjects consumed their habitual diet for 6 weeks.

There were significant decreases in fasting triglycerides, total and LDL cholesterol and oxidized LDL were unaffected, and HDL cholesterol tended to increase.

In subjects with a predominance of small LDL particles pattern B, there were significant increases in mean and peak LDL particle diameter and the percentage of LDL-1.

There were no significant changes in blood lipids in the control group.

The results suggest that a short-term ketogenic diet does not have a deleterious effect on CVD risk profile and may improve the lipid disorders characteristic of atherogenic dyslipidemia.

A Ketogenic Diet Favorably Affects Serum Biomarkers for Cardiovascular Disease in Normal-Weight Men. - 2002

41 overweight or obese people were placed on a very low carbohydrate diet with no limit on caloric intake for 6 months.

- total cholesterol level decreased
- LDL cholesterol level decreased
- triglyceride level decreased
- HDL cholesterol level increased
- cholesterol/HDL cholesterol ratio decreased

Effect of 6-month adherence to a very low carbohydrate diet program. - 2002

20 women completed an 8-week trial that reduced their daily carbohydrate intake from 232 to 71g.

Systolic and diastolic blood pressure decreased, total cholesterol decreased - all of which was accounted for by a decrease in LDL cholesterol with no change in HDL cholesterol. Total triglyceride decreased, and the ratio of triglyceride/HDL also significantly decreased.

Effects of a hypocaloric, low-carbohydrate diet on weight loss, blood lipids, blood pressure, glucose tolerance, and body composition in free-living overweight women. - 2002

10 healthy normolipidemic women were put on a crossover study of a low fat and a very low carbohydrate diet for 4 wk each.

Compared with the low fat diet, the very low carbohydrate diet: increased fasting serum total cholesterol, LDL-C and HDL-C and decreased serum triglyceride, the total cholesterol to HDL ratio and postprandial triglycerides. There were no significant changes in LDL size or markers of inflammation (C-reactive protein, interleukin-6, tumor necrosis factor-α) after the very low carbohydrate diet.

An Isoenergetic Very Low Carbohydrate Diet Improves Serum HDL Cholesterol and triglyceride Concentrations, the Total Cholesterol to HDL Cholesterol Ratio and Postprandial Lipemic Responses Compared with a Low Fat Diet in Normal Weight, Normolipidemic Women. - 2003

24 women with BMI >26 were assigned to either a high carb/moderate protein or moderate carb/high protein diet of 1,700 calories, with ~50g coming from fat in each, therefore only modulating the protein and carbohydrate loads.

The high carb diet followed the USDA Food Pyramid which emphasizes the use of breads, rice, cereals and pasta. The high protein diet substituted foods that emphasized animal proteins including red meats, milk, cheese and eggs, with a requirement for a minimum of seven beef meals each week.

The high protein group had significant reductions in triglycerides and the ratio of TAG/HDL cholesterol.

A reduced ratio of dietary carbohydrate to protein improves body composition and blood lipid profiles during weight loss in adult women. - 2003

Severely obese subjects were randomly assigned to a carbohydrate-restricted or a calorie- and fat-restricted diet.

Subjects on the low carbohydrate diet had greater decreases in triglyceride levels.

A Low-Carbohydrate as Compared with a Low-Fat Diet in Severe Obesity. - 2003

53 obese females were randomized to either a low-fat restricted calorie diet, or a low-carbohydrate unrestricted calorie diet.

Subjects on the very low carbohydrate diet maintained comparable levels of plasma lipids and other cardiovascular risk factors while consuming more than 50% of their calories as fat and 20% as saturated fat.

A Randomized Trial Comparing a Very Low Carbohydrate Diet and a Calorie-Restricted Low Fat Diet on Body Weight and Cardiovascular Risk Factors in Healthy Women. - 2003

A parallel design included either a high-protein diet of meat, poultry, and dairy foods, or a standard-protein diet low in those foods during 12 weeks of energy restriction and 4 weeks of energy balance.

The reduction in serum triglyceride concentrations was significantly greater in the high protein diet group.

Effect of a high-protein, energy-restricted diet on body composition, glycemic control, and lipid concentrations in overweight and obese hyperinsulinemic men and women. - 2003

80 elderly patients put on a low carbohydrate diet of <20g/day experienced a reduction in total cholesterol, LDL cholesterol, triglycerides, LDL particle concentration, small LDL, and large VLDL. However HDL cholesterol and large HDL increased.

Clinical use of a carbohydrate-restricted diet to treat the dyslipidemia of the metabolic syndrome. - 2003

A study group was instructed to consume <20 g of carbohydrate per day for 2 weeks, then <40 g/day for 10 weeks, and to eat low carbohydrate foods according to hunger.

Results were an improvement in non-HDL cholesterol levels and no adverse effects on the lipid profiles.

Effects of a low-carbohydrate diet on weight loss and cardiovascular risk factor in overweight adolescents. - 2003

Obese non-diabetic patients with atherosclerotic cardiovascular disease who had previously been treated with statins were put on a high saturated fat, zero starch diet, which resulted in reduction of triglycerides, VLDL trigs, size and concentration. HDL concentrations remained the same, but HDL and LDL size increased.

No subjects suffered adverse effects on serum lipids.

Effect of a high saturated fat and no-starch diet on serum lipid subfractions in patients with documented atherosclerotic cardiovascular disease. - 2003

83 obese patients with high glucose and cholesterol levels were put on a ketogenic diet for 24 weeks, resulting in reduction of total and LDL cholesterol and triglycerides, whereas HDL cholesterol levels significantly increased.

The changes in the level of urea and creatinine were not statistically significant.

Long-term effects of a ketogenic diet in obese patients. - 2004

Low-carbohydrate diets have been avoided because of the high-fat nature of the diets and the "predicted" associated hypercholesterolemia. However, serum lipids generally improve with the low-carbohydrate diet, especially the triglyceride and HDL measurements.

Replacement of fat with carbohydrates results in significant reductions in HDL cholesterol.

Metabolic Effects of the Very-Low-Carbohydrate Diets: Misunderstood "Villains" of Human Metabolism. - 2004.

15 overweight men consumed a very low-carbohydrate and a low-fat diet for 2 consecutive 6-week periods.

Both diets had the same effect on total cholesterol, insulin, and homeostasis model analysis-insulin resistance (HOMA-IR). Neither diet affected HDL cholesterol or oxidized LDL concentrations.

The low-fat diet was more effective at lowering serum LDL-C, but the very low-carbohydrate diet was more effective at improving characteristics of the metabolic syndrome as shown by a decrease in fasting triglycerides, the trig/HDL-C ratio, postprandial lipemia, serum glucose, an increase in LDL particle size, and also greater weight loss.

Very Low-Carbohydrate and Low-Fat Diets Affect Fasting Lipids and Postprandial Lipemia Differently in Overweight Men. - 2004

A balanced appraisal of the diet–heart hypothesis must recognize the unintended and unanticipated role that the low fat/high carb diet may well have played in the current epidemic of obesity, abnormal lipid patterns, type II diabetes, and the metabolic syndrome. Defense of the diet, because it conforms to current traditional dietary recommendations, by appealing to the authority of its prestigious medical and institutional sponsors or by ignoring an increasingly critical medical literature, is no longer tenable.

The categoric rejection of experience and an increasingly favorable medical literature, though still not conclusive, which suggests that the much-maligned low carb diet may have a favorable impact on obesity, lipid patterns, type II diabetes, and the metabolic syndrome, is also no longer tenable.

The diet-heart hypothesis: a critique. - 2004

120 overweight subjects were assigned either a low carb or low fat diet for 24 weeks.

Compared with recipients of the low-fat diet, recipients of the low-carbohydrate diet had greater decreases in serum triglyceride levels and greater increases in HDL cholesterol levels.

Changes in LDL cholesterol level did not differ statistically.

A Low-Carbohydrate, Ketogenic Diet versus a Low-Fat Diet To Treat Obesity and Hyperlipidemia. A Randomized, Controlled Trial. - 2004

13 healthy moderately overweight women were prescribed an energy restricted diet of either very low-carbohydrate or low-fat.

The low fat diet resulted in HDL-C significantly decreasing whilst fasting glucose, insulin, and insulin resistance were significantly increased. The very low-carbohydrate diet prevented decline in HDL-C and resulted in improved insulin sensitivity.

Comparison of a very low-carbohydrate and low-fat diet on fasting lipids, LDL subclasses, insulin resistance, and postprandial lipemic responses in overweight women. - 2004

132 obese adults assigned either a low carb or low fat restricted calorie diet for 1 year.

The low-carbohydrate diet saw triglyceride levels decreased more and HDL cholesterol levels decreased less. For those with diabetes hemoglobin A1c levels improved more for persons on the low-carbohydrate diet.

These more favorable metabolic responses to a low-carbohydrate diet remained significant after adjustment for weight loss differences.

Changes in other lipids or insulin sensitivity did not differ between groups.

27 premenopausal women and 25 men were assigned to an egg (640mg cholesterol) or placebo diet for 30 days.

Independent of sex, the LDL-1 particle, which is considered to be less atherogenic, was predominant in hyperresponders and this finding was associated with increased cholesterol intake.

Sex, response to cholesterol intake, and diet were not found to affect the susceptibility of LDL to oxidation.

The consumption of a high-cholesterol diet does not negatively influence the atherogenicity of the LDL particle.

High intake of cholesterol results in less atherogenic low-density lipoprotein particles in men and women independent of response classification. - 2004

60 overweight people were assigned to either the US National Cholesterol Education Program (NCEP) diet or a modified low carb (MLC) diet for 12 weeks.

There were no significant differences between the groups for total, low density, and HDL cholesterol, triglycerides, or the proportion of small, dense LDL particles.

There were significantly favorable changes in all lipid levels within the MLC but not within the NCEP group.

The national cholesterol education program diet vs a diet lower in carbohydrates and higher in protein and monounsaturated fat: A randomized trial. - 2004

235 postmenopausal women with established coronary heart disease were studied for 3 years.

A greater saturated fat intake is associated with a smaller decline in mean minimal coronary diameter and less progression of coronary stenosis.

Carbohydrate intake was positively associated with atherosclerotic progression particularly when the glycemic index was high.

Polyunsaturated fat intake was positively associated with progression when replacing other fats but not when replacing carbohydrate or protein.

Dietary fats, carbohydrate, and progression of coronary atherosclerosis in postmenopausal women. - 2004

48 women with BMI >26 were assigned to either a high carb/moderate protein or moderate carb/high protein diet of 1,700 calories.

The high carb diet followed the USDA Food Pyramid which emphasizes restricting fat/cholesterol and the use of breads, rice, cereals and pasta. The moderate carb diet substituted meats, dairy, and eggs.

Subjects in the high carb groups had larger reductions in total and LDL cholesterol, whereas subjects in the moderate carb groups had greater reductions in triglyceride and maintained higher concentrations of HDL cholesterol.

Dietary protein and exercise have additive effects on body composition during weight loss in adult women. - 2005

The most consistent and predictable lipid change with consumption of a very low carb diet is a reduction in triglycerides.

The most dramatic reductions are seen in those with moderate hypertriglyceridemia. A remarkable 79% of the variability in trig response to low carb is explained by pre-diet fasting values, independently of weight loss.

Low-fat diets reduce trigs to a small extent during active weight loss, but increase them when not associated with significant weight loss or combined with exercise.

Modification of Lipoproteins by Very Low-Carbohydrate Diets. - 2005

11 women with a BMI >27 and a clinical diagnosis of PCOS were instructed to limit their carbohydrate intake to 20 grams or less per day for 24 weeks.

Changes in serum lipid levels were not statistically significant. The mean percent change in triglycerides was -25.8%, in HDL was -1.9%, in LDL was +1.6%, and in total cholesterol was +5.4%.

The effects of a low-carbohydrate, ketogenic diet on the polycystic ovary syndrome: a pilot study. - 2005

21 overweight participants with type 2 diabetes maintained a ketogenic diet for 16-weeks with an initial goal of <20g/day of carbohydrate.

Fasting serum triglyceride decreased ~42%, while other serum lipid measurements did not change significantly.

A low-carbohydrate, ketogenic diet to treat type 2 diabetes. - 2005

178 men with a BMI ~29 were put on either a normal high carb (59%), a reduced carb (39%), or moderate carb (26%) diet - with one of the moderate carb groups being assigned low saturated fat, the other high. All diets were restricted by ~1,000 calories, and weight loss over 3 weeks was ~5kg across the board.

After a further 4 weeks of weight stable energy intakes, the 26% carb diets both reduced trigs, apopB, total/HDL cholesterol ratio, and increased LDL sizes. The high sat fat further increased the mass of larger LDLs.

Separate effects of reduced carbohydrate intake and weight loss on atherogenic dyslipidemia. - 2006

Compared to weight loss on a low fat diet, a high saturated fat low carb diet with no weight loss resulted in better improvements in LDL peak size, trigylcerides, HDL, and the ratios total cholesterol/HDL and apoB/ApoA-1.

Carbohydrate restriction alone is significantly better than weight loss on a low fat diet for improving atherogenic dyslipidemia biomarkers.

Low carbohydrate diets improve atherogenic dyslipidemia even in the absence of weight loss. - 2006

The lack of connection between heart disease and egg intake could partially be explained by the fact that dietary cholesterol increases the concentrations of both circulating LDL and HDL cholesterol in hyperresponders.

70% of the population experiences a mild increase or no alterations in plasma cholesterol concentrations.

Egg intake has been shown to shift individuals from the LDL pattern B to pattern A, which is less atherogenic.

Dietary cholesterol provided by eggs and plasma lipoproteins in healthy populations. - 2006

Five trials including a total of 447 individuals assigned randomly to either low carb or low fat diets were meta-analysed.

Triglycerides were reduced and HDL cholesterol values increased on the low carb diets.

Effects of low-carbohydrate vs low-fat diets on weight loss and cardiovascular risk factors: A meta-analysis of randomized controlled trials. - 2006

102 patients with Type 2 diabetes were randomly allocated to a restricted carbohydrate or a reduced-portion, low-fat diet.

Weight loss was greater in the low-carbohydrate group and cholesterol:HDL ratio improved.

Short-term effects of severe dietary carbohydrate-restriction advice in Type 2 diabetes—a randomized controlled trial. - 2006

It is speculated that high saturated fat very low carbohydrate diets have adverse effects on cardiovascular risk but evidence for this in controlled studies is lacking.

83 subjects were assigned to various 1,000 calorie diets, the low carbohydrate diet resulted in similar fat loss as diets low in saturated fat, but was more effective in improving triglycerides, HDL-C, fasting and postprandial glucose, and insulin concentrations.

Comparison of isocaloric very low carbohydrate/high saturated fat and high carbohydrate/low saturated fat diets on body composition and cardiovascular risk. - 2006

29 overweight men consumed an ad libitum low carb diet for 12 weeks.

There were reductions in plasma Lp(a), LDL-C, CRP, and TNF-α.

Effects of a carbohydrate-restricted diet on emerging plasma markers for cardiovascular disease. - 2006

91 patients with non-alcoholic fatty liver disease completed a food frequency questionnaire, 31 had metabolic syndrome.

Patients with metabolic syndrome consumed more carbohydrates and less fat, had a higher HOMA index, scores for steatosis, NASH activity, global NASH score.

Metabolic syndrome is associated with greater histologic severity, higher carbohydrate, and lower fat diet in patients with NAFLD. - 2006

29 overweight men were put on a ketogenic diet for 12 weeks.

Plasma LDL cholesterol, triglycerides, and apolipoproteins were significantly reduced. In contrast plasma HDL-cholesterol concentrations were increased. Changes in plasma TG were positively correlated with reductions in large and medium VLDL particles and negatively correlated with LDL diameter.

Carbohydrate Restriction Alters Lipoprotein Metabolism by Modifying VLDL, LDL, and HDL Subfraction Distribution and Size in Overweight Men. - 2006

66 healthy obese subjects with BMI >30 were put on a ketogenic diet for 56 weeks, about half of which began with high cholesterol.

The level of total cholesterol, LDL cholesterol, triglycerides and blood glucose level decreased significantly, whereas HDL cholesterol increased significantly after the treatment in both groups.

Long term effects of ketogenic diet in obese subjects with high cholesterol level. - 2006

59 subjects were put on a ketogenic diet with nutritional supplementation (including fish, borage and flaxseed oil).

There was a shift from small dense LDL to large buoyant LDL, which could lower cardiovascular disease risk.

Effect of a low-carbohydrate, ketogenic diet program compared to a low-fat diet on fasting lipoprotein subclasses. - 2006

Moderately obese subjects consumed two different low

carb diets as part of a weight loss regimen:

1) a diet high in foods of mammalian origin intended to contain more saturated fat, or

2) a diet high in poultry, fish, and shellfish, intended to contain more PUFA.

Despite high cholesterol and fat intakes, neither diet was associated with significant changes in plasma cholesterol or the plasma lipoprotein cholesterol profile.

Effects of low carbohydrate diets high in red meats or poultry, fish and shellfish on plasma lipids and weight loss. - 2007

Outpatient obesity studies found a consistent reduction in fasting triglycerides and a fairly consistent increase in HDL cholesterol, but little change in total or LDL cholesterol in low carb groups.

Low-carbohydrate nutrition and metabolism. - 2007

64 obese diabetic subjects on a ketogenic diet for 56 weeks underwent a significant decrease in blood glucose, total cholesterol, LDL-cholesterol, triglycerides, and urea. The level of HDL-cholesterol increased significantly.

Beneficial effects of ketogenic diet in obese diabetic subjects. - 2007

311 obese women were assigned one of 4 weight-loss diets representing a spectrum of low to high carbohydrate intake for effects on weight loss and related metabolic

variables over 12 months.

Subjects assigned to follow the Atkins diet, which had the lowest carbohydrate intake, experienced more favorable overall metabolic effects than those assigned to follow the Zone, Ornish, or LEARN diets.

Comparison of the atkins, zone, ornish, and learn diets for change in weight and related risk factors among overweight premenopausal women: The a to z weight loss study: a randomized trial. - 2007

Rats were fed a normal, high carbohydrate, or ketogenic diet for 19 weeks.

Electron microscopes demonstrate a decrease in the number of mitochondria when fed a high carbohydrate diet and an increase in those fed a ketogenic diet.

Keto subjects had a remarkable tolerance to restriction of blood supply to the heart, and a faster recovery of cardiac function following blood-restricted damage.

Low carbohydrate ketogenic diet enhances cardiac tolerance to global ischaemia. - 2007

39 subjects were randomized to an energy restricted diet which was either low fat or ketogenic. Blood pH decreased mildly in both groups.

Acid-base analysis of individuals following two weight loss diets. - 2007

88 obese adults were put on an either very low

carb/high fat or high carb/low fat diet for 24 weeks, both with energy restricted by 30%.

The low carb group had greater decreases in triglycerides and increases in HDL cholesterol. LDL cholesterol decreased in the high carb diet but remained unchanged in the low carb diet. There was no correlation between the change in LDL-C and the change in saturated fat intake or weight loss.

ApoB levels did not change significantly in either diet group, suggesting that atherogenicity did not change regardless of saturated fat intake or in the absence of an expected reduction in LDL-C with weight loss in the low carb diet. A meta-analysis showed that apoB levels were not affected by the replacement of dietary carbohydrate with saturated fat.

A high saturated fat intake in the context of carbohydrate-restriction has been shown to increase larger LDL particles rather than smaller atherogenic LDL particles.

The very low carb/high fat diet may confer the greatest clinical benefits in patients who present with hypertriglyceridemia, low HDL levels, abdominal adiposity, and insulin resistance.

Metabolic Effects of Weight Loss on a Very-Low-Carbohydrate Diet Compared With an Isocaloric High-Carbohydrate Diet in Abdominally Obese Subjects. - 2008

Obese children between 6 and 12 years old were put on a diet restricted in carbs to <30g but otherwise unrestricted in fat and protein.

Cholesterol and triglycerides were reduced significantly

after 10 weeks.

Unlimited energy, restricted carbohydrate diet improves lipid parameters in
obese children - 2008

Overweight men and women with atherogenic dyslipidemia consumed ad libitum diets very low in carbohydrate or low in fat for 12 weeks.

Both diets significantly decreased the concentration of several serum inflammatory markers, but there was an overall greater anti-inflammatory effect associated with the low carb diet.

Comparison of low fat and low carbohydrate diets on circulating fatty acid
composition and markers of inflammation. - 2008

99 obese subjects were put on a weight loss diet of either very-low-carbohydrate high-saturated-fat, or high-carbohydrate low-saturated-fat, for 8 weeks.

HDL cholesterol did not change with the high carb group, but increased with low carb. Triglycerides decreased overall, to a greater extent with the low carb diet.

A very-low-carbohydrate high fat diet with significant portion as saturated fat diet not impair brachial artery flow-mediated dilatation.

Effects of weight loss from a very-low-carbohydrate diet on endothelial
function and markers of cardiovascular disease risk in subjects with
abdominal obesity. - 2008

Carbohydrate, directly or indirectly through the effect of insulin, controls the disposition of excess dietary nutrients. Dietary carbohydrate modulates lipolysis, lipoprotein assembly and processing and affects the relation between dietary intake of saturated fat intake and circulating levels.

Low-carbohydrate diet trials have shown reduced cardiovascular risk through improvement in hepatic, intravascular, and peripheral processing of lipoproteins, alterations in fatty acid composition, and reductions in other cardiovascular risk factors, notably inflammation.

The data suggest that some form of carbohydrate restriction is a candidate to be the preferred dietary strategy for cardiovascular health beyond weight regulation.

Dietary carbohydrate restriction induces a unique metabolic state positively affecting atherogenic dyslipidemia, fatty acid partitioning, and metabolic syndrome. - 2008

55 people of ~33 BMI were put on diets restricted by ~500 calories for 4 months, of either 1.6g/kg protein and <170g carbohydrate, or 0.8g/kg protein and >220g carbohydrate.

There was a trend for lower carb to favor reductions in triglyceride and increases in HDL-C.

Moderate carbohydrate, moderate protein weight loss diet reduces cardiovascular disease risk compared to high carbohydrate, low protein diet in obese adults: A randomized clinical trial. - 2008

28 overweight men consumed an ad libitum low carb diet for 12 weeks, and randomly assigned to consume eggs as well.

Subjects in the egg group decreased plasma CRP and increased plasma adiponectin compared to the others. These findings indicate that eggs make a significant contribution to the anti-inflammatory effects of carb restriction, possibly due to the presence of cholesterol, which increases HDL-C and to the antioxidant lutein which modulates certain inflammatory responses.

Eggs modulate the inflammatory response to carbohydrate restricted diets in overweight men. - 2008

31 obese subjects undertook a so-called "Spanish Ketogenic Mediterranean Diet" which is based on fish, green veggies and salads, virgin olive oil, and moderate red wine intake. It is an unlimited calorie diet.

After 3 months there was a significant improvement in all features of metabolic syndrome and cardiovascular risk markers, such as:

- systolic and diastolic blood pressure reduced
- total cholesterol (~208 → ~186)
- triacylglicerols (~halved)
- glucose (~110 → ~93)
- LDL-C (~114 → ~106)
- HDL-C was increased

Spanish Ketogenic Mediterranean diet: a healthy cardiovascular diet for weight loss. - 2008

31 healthy people with an average age of ~52 were on a low carb high fat diet for at least 1 year, most more than 3 years, with an average of 4 years adherence.

The longer the adherence to the diet the lower the blood pressure and BMI.

Averages for total cholesterol were ~270, LDL-C ~180, HDL-C ~70, triglycerides ~93, and the trig:HDL ratio 1.4.

In most subjects glucose, insulin, glucagon, cortisol, homocysteine, glycerol, and C-reactive protein were within reference ranges.

Long-term consumption of a carbohydrate-restricted diet does not induce deleterious metabolic effects. - 2008

Subjects were put on a diet restricted by ~500 calories comprised of either 1.6g/kg of protein and <170g of carbohydrates, or 0.8g/kg of protein and >220g of carbs.

The high carb diet reduced total and LDL cholesterol more at 4 months, but the effect did not remain at 12 months. Lower carb group had sustained favorable effects on trigs, HDL cholesterol, and TAG:HDL-C ratio compared with high carb at 4 and 12 months.

A moderate-protein diet produces sustained weight loss and long-term changes in body composition and blood lipids in obese adults. - 2009

This systematic review included all known RCTs of low-carb diets vs the low-fat/high-carb diet from 2000 to 2007. Factors including weight, cholesterol, blood pressure and glycemic control were evaluated, as these are important in weight loss and cardiovascular disease risk.

Evidence from this systematic review demonstrates that low carb diets are more effective at 6 months and are as effective, if not more, as low fat diets in reducing weight and cardiovascular disease risk up to 1 year.

Systematic review of randomized controlled trials of low-carbohydrate vs. low-fat/low-calorie diets in the management of obesity and its comorbidities. - 2009

200 overweight subjects were randomly assigned to a conventional high-carb or a moderate-carb diet.

Triglycerides, HDL-cholesterol, waist circumference and systolic blood pressure all improved more in the lower carb group.

A randomized controlled trial on the efficacy of carbohydrate-reduced or fat-reduced diets in patients attending a telemedically guided weight loss program. - 2009

39 participants with metabolic syndrome followed a lowish-carb diet by eliminating rice and bread, reducing yogurt and milk, and consuming only 1 fruit per day.

After 6 weeks plasma triglycerides dropped ~39%, and there were significant decreases in LDL cholesterol, blood pressure, glucose, insulin, and inflammatory markers, and increases in adiponectin also occurred.

Carbohydrate Restriction, as a First-Line Dietary Intervention, Effectively Reduces Biomarkers of Metabolic Syndrome in Emirati Adults. - 2009

69 participants (of 118, high attrition) completed a year of either very low carb or a standard diet, both of similar moderately restricted calories.

The low carb group had greater decreases in triglycerides, increases in HDL and LDL cholesterol.

Long-term effects of a very-low-carbohydrate weight loss diet compared with an isocaloric low-fat diet after 12 mo. - 2009

Subjects with atherogenic dyslipidemia were examined on a 12-week study comparing two ~1,500 kcal diets, a carbohydrate-restricted and a low-fat diet.

Both interventions led to improvements in several metabolic markers, but subjects following the low carb diet experienced:

- reduced glucose (−12%)
- reduced insulin (−50%)
- insulin sensitivity (−55%)
- triglyceride (−51%)
- HDL-C (13%)
- total cholesterol/HDL-C ratio (−14%)

Despite a threefold higher intake of dietary saturated fat during the carbohydrate restriction, saturated fatty acids in triglyceride and cholesteryl ester were significantly decreased, as was palmitoleic acid, an endogenous marker of lipogenesis, compared to subjects consuming the low fat diet.

Carbohydrate Restriction has a More Favorable Impact on the Metabolic Syndrome than a Low Fat Diet. - 2009

Ketogenic mice normalized fasting glycemia and substantially reduced insulin and lipid levels in the absence of weight loss.

Ketogenic feeding was associated with significant increases in lipid oxidative genes and reduced expression of lipid synthetic genes, including stearoyl-coenzyme A desaturase 1, but no change in expression of inflammatory markers.

A very low carbohydrate ketogenic diet improves glucose tolerance in ob/ob mice independently of weight loss. - 2009

A meta-analysis of prospective epidemiologic studies showed that there is no significant evidence for concluding that dietary saturated fat is associated with an increased risk of CHD or CVD. More data are needed to elucidate whether CVD risks are likely to be influenced by the specific nutrients used to replace saturated fat.

Meta-analysis of prospective cohort studies evaluating the association of saturated fat with cardiovascular disease. - 2010

Carbohydrate restriction favorably alters VLDL metabolism and apolipoprotein concentrations, while the components of the egg yolk favor the formation of larger LDL and HDL leading to an increase in plasma lutein and zeaxanthin. [anti-oxidants]

Eggs distinctly modulate plasma carotenoid and lipoprotein subclasses in adult men following a carbohydrate-restricted diet. - 2010

After 5 weeks on a normal high carb diet, subjects with untreated type 2 diabetes followed a moderately reduced carbohydrate diet. After 10 weeks diabetic biomarkers had improved significantly, with no adverse effects on serum lipids, blood pressure, hormones, or kidney function.

Further decrease in glycated hemoglobin following ingestion of a LoBAG30 diet for 10 weeks compared to 5 weeks in people with untreated type 2 diabetes. - 2010

21 studies with 5–23 years of follow-up data of 347,747 subjects, demonstrated 11,006 developed CHD or stroke.

Intake of saturated fat was not associated with an increased risk of CHD, stroke, or CVD.

Meta-analysis of prospective cohort studies evaluating the association of saturated fat with cardiovascular disease. - 2010

Prospective epidemiologic studies have generated mixed results regarding the association between saturated fatty acid intake and risk of ischemic heart disease and stroke.

The Japan Collaborative Cohort Study for Evaluation of Cancer Risk comprised 58,453 Japanese men and women, saturated fat intake was inversely associated with mortality from stroke, and no associations were observed between saturated fat intake and mortality from cerebral hemorrhage or heart disease.

Dietary intake of saturated fatty acids and mortality from cardiovascular disease in Japanese: the Japan Collaborative Cohort Study for Evaluation

Obese subjects without diabetes or dyslipidemia were put on either an unlimited calorie low-carbohydrate or low-fat diet of limited energy intake. Low carbers were at 20g/d for 3 months and then increased carbohydrate intake 5g/d per wk until a stable and desired weight was achieved.

During the first 6 months the low-carbohydrate diet group had greater reductions in diastolic blood pressure, triglyceride levels, and VLDL cholesterol levels, lesser reductions in LDL cholesterol levels, and greater increases in HDL cholesterol levels at all time points.

Weight and metabolic outcomes after 2 years on a low-carbohydrate versus low-fat diet: a randomized trial. - 2010

22 obese subjects with metabolic syndrome under free-living conditions followed the Spanish Ketogenic Mediterranean Diet for 3 months.

There was significant improvement in all parameters, LDL cholesterol, body weight, BMI, waist circumference, fasting glucose, triglycerides, HDL cholesterol, and blood pressure.

A pilot study of the Spanish Ketogenic Mediterranean Diet: an effective therapy for the metabolic syndrome. 2011

14 obese men who were put on a Spanish Ketogenic Mediterranean Diet for 12 weeks.

There was a significant improvement in LDL-cholesterol, fasting plasma glucose, triglycerides, HDL-cholesterol, systolic blood pressure, and diastolic blood pressure.

The effect of the Spanish Ketogenic Mediterranean Diet on nonalcoholic fatty liver disease: a pilot study - 2011

106 subjects were put on a modified ketogenic diet based on green vegetables, olive oil, fish and meat plus dishes composed of high quality protein and virtually zero carbohydrate, with the addition of some herbal extracts. Calories in the diet were unlimited.

After 6 weeks there was a significant reduction in total cholesterol, LDL-C, triglycerides, and blood glucose. HDL-C increased significantly.

There were no significant changes in BUN, ALT, AST, GGT and blood creatinine.

Effect of ketogenic mediterranean diet with phytoextracts and low carbohydrates/high-protein meals on weight, cardiovascular risk factors, body composition and diet compliance in Italian council employees. - 2011

Adiponectin is an adipose-derived protein with beneficial metabolic effects. 81 obese women in 2 cohorts (of 6 and 4 months) were randomized to a low-fat or a low-carbohydrate diet.

Adiponectin increased significantly more in the low carb group.

Adiponectin changes in relation to the macronutrient composition of a weight-loss diet. - 2011

58 obese children were placed on either a ketogenic or low calorie diet for 6 months. Both groups significantly reduced their weight, fasting insulin, and HOMA-IR, but the differences were greater in the ketogenic group. Both groups increased insulin sensitivity significantly, but only the ketogenic group increased adiponectin significantly.

Metabolic impact of a ketogenic diet compared to a hypocaloric diet in obese children and adolescents. - 2012

23 randomized controlled trials with a total of 2,788 participants between 1966 and 2011 were included in a meta-analysis, anything below 45% carbohydrate considered to be "low carb" and compared with anything below 30% fat, so whilst nowhere near ketogenic nor even low carb, the diets are more restricted in carbohydrates and higher in fat than those being compared.

Persons on lower-carbohydrate diets experienced a slightly but statistically significantly lower reduction in total cholesterol and LDL-C, but a greater increase in HDL-C and a greater decrease in triglycerides.

These findings suggest that reduced carb/increased fat diets are at least as effective as low-fat diets at improving metabolic risk factors.

Effects of low-carbohydrate diets versus low-fat diets on metabolic risk factors: a meta-analysis of randomized controlled clinical trials. - 2012

Treatment of cells in mice with ketone bodies conferred substantial protection against oxidative stress.

Replacing saturated fats with monounsaturated fat or carbohydrates in healthy subjects does not affect vascular function.

SFAs do not impair endothelial function and arterial stiffness. - 2013

The present meta-analysis aimed to investigate whether individuals assigned to a ketogenic diet achieve better long-term cardiovascular risk factor management when compared with individuals assigned to a conventional low-fat diet.

Patients assigned to a very-low-carbohydrate ketogenic diet had significantly decreased triglyceride and diastolic blood pressure, and significantly increased HDL cholesterol and LDL cholesterol compared with patients on a low fat diet.

There was no significant difference between treatment groups in changes in systolic blood pressure, fasting blood glucose, insulin, HbA1c and C-reactive protein.

Very-low-carbohydrate ketogenic diet v. low-fat diet for long-term weight loss: a meta-analysis of randomised controlled trials. - 2013

Overweight type-2 diabetes patients without overt heart disease were studied in a parallel and partial cross-over of low fat and low carb diets.

Low carb considerably improved insulin resistance, fasting and postmeal triglycerides, blood pressure, post-prandial intact proinsulin and diastolic cardiac function. None of these variables changed on low fat.

Low-carbohydrate/high-protein diet improves diastolic cardiac function and the metabolic syndrome in overweight-obese patients with type 2 diabetes.

- 2014

The inhibitory effect of ketone bodies on advanced glycation end-products was studied after 35 days of incubation. The measurements of glycated HSA by glucose in the presence of ketones indicate a decrease in AGEs formation.

The concentration of ketones used in this study is in accordance with the concentration detected in the body of individuals post fasting and prolonged exercises, or on a ketogenic diet.

Inhibition of fluorescent advanced glycation end products (AGEs) of human serum albumin upon incubation with 3-β-hydroxybutyrate. - 2014

Diabetes

The treatment of diabetes mellitus has been very greatly improved in the recent past, the urine of the severest diabetics can be made sugar free by sufficiently prolonged starvation and will remain sugar free if the total energy intake is kept sufficiently small.

It has been the general custom to make up the diet largely of protein, because of the undoubted desirability of omitting carbohydrates, and because of the almost universal fear of precipitating a dangerous acidosis by allowing more than a minimum of fat.

The dilemma [hyperglycaemia OR low energy] can be avoided if the diabetic can safely be given enough calories to maintain metabolic equilibrium, without producing acidosis.

Since carbohydrate cannot be used, we have dared to ignore the belief concerning the danger of fat in the diet of diabetics, and have investigated in the clinic the effect of a diet whose energy comes largely from fat.

The use of a high fat diet in the treatment of diabetes mellitus: First paper
- 1920

The advantages of the use of a high fat diet in the treatment of diabetes mellitus were discussed in outline previously.

The results of an investigation of the effect of a diet whose energy came largely from fat were reported briefly, to which was added sufficient protein to maintain nitrogen balance and the minimal carbohydrate necessitated in making up a diet that a human being can eat over a long period of time.

It was shown that with such a diet, glycosuria was avoided in severe diabetics, and that acidosis was not produced.

The use of a high fat diet in the treatment of diabetes mellitus: Second paper: blood sugar. - 1921

Objections to the use of a diet high in protein for diabetics fall into 3 main groups:

- protein is said to exert a specific action which interferes with the mechanism of sugar utilization;
- the dynamic effect of protein in increasing heat production was wasteful in terms of total energy expenditure and as such should be minimized;
- protein constituted a large source of endogenous glucose and therefore should be carefully curtailed in the diabetic diet.

The latter is the only one that has in any measure stood the test of time as far as practical diabetic management is concerned, however when an equivalent amount of glucose is derived from protein the blood sugar curve remains flat.

THE GLYCEMIC RESPONSE TO ISOGLUCOGENIC QUANTITIES OF PROTEIN AND CARBOHYDRATE. - 1936

Before the discovery of insulin the best results for treatment of diabetes were obtained with dietary methods.

It was shown in 1770 that the sweet taste of the urine in diabetes - first pointed out 100 years earlier - was due to the presence of sugar, the origin was found to be starch converted to sugar in the intestines. On this theoretical basis it was pertinent to treat diabetics with an almost exclusive meat diet.

The guiding principle in the modern pre-insulin methods of treatment was to spare the disturbed carbohydrate metabolism by reducing the carbohydrate content of the food. During this period the patients usually received fairly abundant quantities of a diet poor in carbohydrates, and rich in proteins and fat.

Diet and the Genesis of Diabetes Mellitus - 1947

Patients with diabetes were put on diets in a random crossover design of 15 days each, one low fat high carb resembling recommendations made by the American Diabetes Association, the other moderate fat and carbohydrate.

In the ADA diet incremental glucose and insulin responses from 8 a.m. to 4 p.m. were higher and mean 24-hour urine glucose excretion was significantly greater. Also fasting and postprandial triglyceride levels were increased, HDL-C was reduced, and the HDL/LDL cholesterol ratio fell.

Deleterious metabolic effects of high-carbohydrate, sucrose-containing diets in patients with non-insulin-dependent diabetes mellitus. - 1987

10 diabetic patients were randomly assigned in crossover design a diet of either low fat high carb or

moderate fat moderate carb each for 28 days.

The moderate diet resulted in lower glucose and reduced insulin requirements.

Comparison of a High-Carbohydrate Diet with a High-Monounsaturated-Fat Diet in Patients with Non-Insulin-Dependent Diabetes Mellitus. - 1988

Subjects were placed on diets of either low fat high carb or moderate fat and carb, consumed in random order for 6 weeks in a crossover design.

On the higher carb diet glucose and insulin were significantly elevated throughout the day, and 24-h urinary glucose excretion more than doubled.

Persistence of Hypertriglyceridemic Effect of Low-Fat High-Carbohydrate Diets in NIDDM Patients. - 1989

10 non-insulin-dependent diabetic patients aged ~52 with a BMI ~26.7 who were being treated with diet alone or with diet plus glibenclamide were randomly assigned to a 15-day period of either a moderate carb moderate fat diet high in MUFA or a high carb low fat diet and were then crossed-over to the other diet.

The moderate carb diet saw a decrease in both postprandial glucose and plasma insulin, as well as reduced triglyceride levels.

A high-monounsaturated-fat/low-carbohydrate diet improves peripheral insulin sensitivity in non-insulin-dependent diabetic patients. - 1992

42 diabetic patients were put on a low fat high carb or moderate fat and carb diet for 6 weeks one after the other.

The high carb diet increased glucose levels and hyperinsulinemia.

Effects of varying carbohydrate content of diet in patients with non—insulin-dependent diabetes mellitus. - 1994

Women with gestational diabetes on either a high or moderate carb diet were studied.

In the lower-carbohydrate group there were significant reductions in postprandial glucose, and fewer subjects required the addition of insulin for glucose control.

The effects of carbohydrate restriction in patients with diet-controlled gestational diabetes. - 1998

Subjects with type 2 diabetes were placed on a 25% carbohydrate diet for 8 weeks then switched to a 55% carbohydrate diet.

After the lower carb diet subjects showed significantly improved fasting glucose and hemoglobin A1c levels, but when switched to the high carbohydrate diet the hemoglobin A1c rose significantly.

Utility of a short-term 25% carbohydrate diet on improving glycemic control in type 2 diabetes mellitus. - 1998

8 men were randomized on a 5-week crossover between a normal high carb and a low carb diet.

The mean 24h integrated serum glucose at the end of the control diet was 198, at the end of the low carb diet it was 126. Glycohemoglobin dropped from ~9.8 to ~7.6, and was still decreasing at the end. Insulin was decreased, and glucagon was increased.

Effect of a high-protein, low-carbohydrate diet on blood glucose control in people with type 2 diabetes. - 2004

In a small group of obese patients with type 2 diabetes, a low-carbohydrate diet followed for 2 weeks resulted in much improved 24-hour blood glucose profiles, insulin sensitivity, and hemoglobin A1c. Reduced glucose also called for a decrease in diabetes medication in 5 of the 10 patients.

Effect of a low-carbohydrate diet on appetite, blood glucose levels, and insulin resistance in obese patients with type 2 diabetes. - 2005

Prior to the advent of exogenous insulin for the treatment of diabetes mellitus in the 1920's, the mainstay of therapy was dietary modification. Diet recommendations in that era consisted of "meats, poultry, game, fish, clear soups, gelatin, eggs, butter, olive oil, coffee, tea" and contained approximately 5% of energy from carbohydrates, 20% from protein, and 75% from fat.

In this study the ketogenic diet had positive effects on body weight, waist measurement, serum triglycerides, and glycemic control in a cohort of 21 participants with type 2 diabetes who completed the intervention over 16 weeks.

Most impressive is that improvement in hemoglobin A1c was observed despite a small sample size and short duration of follow-up, and this improvement in glycemic control occurred while diabetes medications were reduced substantially in many participants.

A low-carbohydrate, ketogenic diet to treat type 2 diabetes. - 2005

Before the discovery of insulin, one of the most common dietary treatments of diabetes mellitus was a high-fat, low-carbohydrate diet.

A review of case histories shows that a 70% fat, 8% carbohydrate diet could eliminate glycosuria among hospitalized patients.

Dietary treatment of diabetes mellitus in the pre-insulin era (1914-1922) - 2006

Before the discovery of insulin, the removal of high-glycemic carbohydrates such as sugar and flour from the diets of diabetics was found to be a successful method of controlling glycosuria.

An analysis of the pattern of food consumption during the more recent obesity and diabetes epidemic found that the increase in calories was almost entirely due to an increase in carbohydrate

Low-carbohydrate nutrition and metabolism. - 2007

64 obese diabetic subjects were put on a ketogenic diet and monitored for 56 weeks, during which a significant decrease in body weight, body mass index, the level of blood glucose, total cholesterol, LDL-cholesterol, triglycerides, and urea was expressed. The level of HDL-cholesterol increased significantly.

These changes were more significant in subjects with high blood glucose level as compared to those with normal blood glucose level.

Beneficial effects of ketogenic diet in obese diabetic subjects. - 2007

13 type-2 diabetic and non-diabetic subjects were randomly allocated to either a low-carbohydrate diet or a healthy-eating diet following Diabetes UK nutritional recommendations for 3 months.

Weight loss was greater in the low-carbohydrate group, with no difference in changes in HbA1c, ketone or lipid levels.

A low-carbohydrate diet is more effective in reducing body weight than healthy eating in both diabetic and non-diabetic subjects. - 2007

During 20 years of follow-up, 4,670 cases of type 2 diabetes in women were documented.

A higher dietary glycemic load was strongly associated with an increased risk of diabetes, a higher carbohydrate consumption was also associated with an increased risk.

These data suggest that diets lower in carbohydrate and higher in fat and protein do not increase the risk of type 2 diabetes in women.

13 short term studies were included in a meta analysis on restricted carbohydrate diets effects on patients with type 2 diabetes.

Hemoglobin A1c, fasting glucose, and some lipid fractions (triglycerides) improved with lower carbohydrate-content diets.

Restricted-carbohydrate diets in patients with type 2 diabetes: a meta-analysis. - 2008

Dietary carbohydrate restriction in the treatment of diabetes is based on an underlying principle of controlling chronic hyperglycemia and therefore hyperinsulinemia. It has generally been opposed by health agencies because of concern that carbohydrate will be replaced by fat, particularly saturated fat.

Removing the barrier of concern about dietary fat makes carbohydrate restriction a reasonable, if not the preferred method for treating type 2 diabetes, considering the ability of low carbohydrate diets to improve glycemic control, hemoglobin A1C, and to reduce medication.

Carbohydrate restriction as the default treatment for type 2 diabetes and metabolic syndrome. - 2008

8 men with untreated type 2 diabetes were put on a moderate carbohydrate weight-maintenance diet for 5

weeks.

Fasting glucose concentration decreased by ~40%; 24h glucose area response decreased by ~45%. Insulin did not change. Mean total glycohaemoglobin decreased by ~1.7, and was still decreasing linearly at 5 weeks.

Effect of the LoBAG30 diet on blood glucose control in people with type 2 diabetes. - 2008

Subjects with type 2 diabetes on a low carbohydrate diet after 6 months had lost ~11kg. In a follow-up after the intervention period at 22 months, mean bodyweight had increased by ~2.7kg, and at 44 months average weight has increased another ~1kg.

The initial mean HbA1c was ~8.0, after 6, 12 and 22 months, HbA1c was ~6.1, ~7.0, and ~6.9 respectively. After 44 months mean HbA1c is ~6.8.

Low-carbohydrate diet in type 2 diabetes: stable improvement of bodyweight and glycemic control during 44 months follow-up. - 2008

In the early 20th century, before any medications were available for the treatment of diabetes mellitus, experts recommended dietary carbohydrate-restriction.

The dietary recommendation for diabetes in a prominent internal medicine textbook from 1923 was 75% fat, 17% protein, 6% alcohol and only 2% carbohydrate.

After the discovery of insulin and oral hypoglycemic medications, experts gradually changed the dietary recommendations to include more carbohydrate intake because most experts reasoned that the medications could be used to keep the glucose in control.

Has carbohydrate-restriction been forgotten as a treatment for diabetes mellitus? A perspective on the ACCORD study design. - 2008

Subjects with obesity and type 2 diabetes were randomized to either a low-carbohydrate, ketogenic diet or a low-glycemic, reduced-calorie diet.

Both interventions led to improvements in hemoglobin A1c, fasting glucose, fasting insulin, and weight loss. The ketogenic group had greater improvements in hemoglobin A1c, body weight, and HDL cholesterol compared to the low glycemic group. Diabetes medications were reduced or eliminated in 95.2% of ketogenic dieters vs. 62% of low glycemic participants.

Lifestyle modification using low carbohydrate interventions is effective for improving and reversing type 2 diabetes.

The effect of a low-carbohydrate, ketogenic diet versus a low-glycemic index diet on glycemic control in type 2 diabetes mellitus. - 2008

In a retrospective review of patients attending an outpatient metabolic management program 31 patients aged ~58 were prescribed a high fat low carb diet.

Along with many other metabolic improvements, insulin and fasting glucose levels were significantly reduced.

Clinical Experience of a Diet Designed to Reduce Aging. - 2009

This study compared the effects of a eucaloric high carb/low fat versus low carbohydrate/high fat (monounsaturated) on postmeal triglycerideconcentrations and other cardiovascular disease risk factors in nonobese subjects with type 1 diabetes with good glycemic control.

There were no significant differences between groups other than decreased plasminogen activator inhibitor 1 levels, weight gain, and lower triglycerides in the low carb group.

Effects of a Diet Higher in Carbohydrate/Lower in Fat Versus Lower in Carbohydrate/Higher in Monounsaturated Fat on Postmeal Triglyceride Concentrations and Other Cardiovascular Risk Factors in Type 1 Diabetes.

\- 2009

33 outpatients with severe type 2 diabetes and HbA1c levels of ~10.9% were instructed to follow a moderate carbohydrate diet for 6 months.

HbA1c levels decreased sharply to ~7.8% within 3 months and to ~7.4% at 6 months.

Effects of a low-carbohydrate diet on glycemic control in outpatients with severe type 2 diabetes. - 2009

Adult rats were divided into 3 groups: normal diet, keto, and high-carbohydrate diet. Diabetes was induced by injection.

The results showed that a ketogenic diet was effective in bringing blood glucose level close to normal, and has a significant beneficial effect in ameliorating the diabetic state.

Therapeutic role of low-carbohydrate ketogenic diet in diabetes. - 2009

After 5 weeks on a normal high carb diet, subjects with untreated type 2 diabetes followed a moderate carbohydrate diet. After 5 weeks it resulted in a significant decrease in glycated hemoglobin, and both the fasting glucose and postprandial glucose area were decreased.

After a further 5 weeks on the diet these parameters continued to improve linearly and was still improving, with no adverse effects on serum lipids, blood pressure, hormones, or kidney function.

Further decrease in glycated hemoglobin following ingestion of a LoBAG30 diet for 10 weeks compared to 5 weeks in people with untreated type 2 diabetes. - 2010

15 months of follow-up of a 3.5 year old girl with diabetes type 1 demonstrated an improved activity level and significant developmental achievements, glycosylated hemoglobin (HbA1c) levels improved, and glycemic control was excellent, without severe side effects.

During the 15-month observation period, no severe hypoglycemia or ketoacidosis occurred, no deficit in selenium and zinc levels was present, and uric acids were normal.

Our experience indicates that type 1 diabetes does not preclude the use of the ketogenic diet.

Type 1 diabetes and epilepsy: efficacy and safety of the ketogenic diet. - 2010

65 participants with type 2 diabetes or impaired glucose tolerance were randomised to a high protein diet either high or low in cholesterol.

These results suggest that a high-protein energy-restricted diet high in cholesterol from eggs improved glycaemic and lipid profiles, blood pressure and apo-B in individuals with type 2 diabetes.

Egg consumption as part of an energy-restricted high-protein diet improves blood lipid and blood glucose profiles in individuals with type 2 diabetes. - 2011

Intensive insulin therapy and protein restriction delay the development of nephropathy (kidney disease) in a variety of conditions, but few interventions are known to reverse nephropathy.

In mouse models for both Type 1 and Type 2 diabetes, diabetic nephropathy was allowed to develop, then half the mice were switched to a ketogenic diet. After 8 weeks it was completely reversed.

Reversal of Diabetic Nephropathy by a Ketogenic Diet. - 2011

Rats were fed ad libitum for 8 weeks on either a normal diet, a high carb diet, or a ketogenic diet, then injected with streptozotocin - a chemical which is toxic to insulin-producing beta cells in the pancreas, thus inducing diabetes.

Blood glucose, food intake, water intake, urine output, and weight gain were significantly increased in all but the ketogenic rats.

A substantial decrease in the number of beta cells was noticed in all injected rats except for the ketogenic subjects.

Low carbohydrate ketogenic diet prevents the induction of diabetes using streptozotocin in rats. - 2011

363 overweight and obese people were put on a 24-wk diet intervention trial, free to choose either a low calorie or ketogenic diet. 102 of them with type 2 diabetes.

Both diets had beneficial effects on all the parameters examined. These changes were more significant in subjects who were on the ketogenic diet as compared with those restricting calories.

The initial dose of some antidiabetic medications was decreased to half and some were discontinued at the beginning of the dietary program in the ketogenic group.

Effect of low-calorie versus low-carbohydrate ketogenic diet in type 2 diabetes. - 2012

Accumulating evidence suggests that low-carbohydrate, high-fat diets are safe and effective to reduce glycemia in diabetic patients without producing significant cardiovascular risks.

Treatment of diabetes and diabetic complications with a ketogenic diet - 2013

The aim of this study was to examine the effects of a

non-calorie-restricted, low-carbohydrate diet in Japanese patients unable to adhere to a calorie-restricted diet.

The HbA1c levels decreased significantly from baseline to 6 months in the low-carbohydrate diet group but not in the calorie-restricted group.

The patients in the former group also experienced improvements in their triglyceride levels, without experiencing any major adverse effects or a decline in the quality of life.

A non-calorie-restricted low-carbohydrate diet is effective as an alternative therapy for patients with type 2 diabetes. - 2014

Subjects were assigned to either a medium carb/low fat/calorie restricted (MCCR) diet as specified by the American Diabetes Association, or an unrestricted ketogenic diet.

After 3 months HbA1c level was unchanged in the MCCR diet group, while it decreased in the keto group. 44% of the keto subjects discontinued one or more diabetes medications, compared to 11% of the MCCR group.

A Randomized Pilot Trial of a Moderate Carbohydrate Diet Compared to a Very Low Carbohydrate Diet in Overweight or Obese Individuals with Type 2 Diabetes Mellitus or Prediabetes. - 2014

Weight Loss

A diet consisting essentially of protein and fat is ketogenic. Ketogenesis, it appears, is the normal mechanism by which the organism is enabled to utilize fat in much larger quantities than it otherwise could.

In the practical use of this method a minimum of 8 ounces (226g) of meat has been recommended for each of the 3 meals of the day; and to emphasize that fat, as well as lean, is to be eaten, one part of fat to 3 parts of lean meat has been suggested as the proper proportion. This is the general proportion adopted by choice when an exclusive meat diet has been followed.

A DIET FOR OBESITY

With this diet you follow a definite routine which is as important as the diet itself. Have a regular hour for going to bed. Set your alarm clock for eight hours sleep, never a minute more than that, and allow time for a 30-minute walk before breakfast. It is not necessary to walk fast, but it is necessary to walk the full 30 minutes regularly.

Breakfast, lunch, and dinner are all the same type. You eat 3 big meals a day and lose seven pounds of excess weight a month.

First course of each meal: One-half pound or more of fresh meat with the fat.

This part of the diet is unlimited. You can eat as much as you want.

The proper proportion is three parts of lean to one part fat. Most of the meat you buy is not fat enough, so get extra beef kidney fat, slice and fry it to make up the proper proportion. Good meats are roast beef, steak, roast lamb, lamb chops, stewed beef, fresh pork, and pork chops. Hamburger is all right if you grind it yourself just before it is cooked. Season the meat with black pepper before it is cooked or use paprika, celery seed, lemon, chopped parsley, or celery tops, or use other flavoring which does not contain salt.

Do not use the least particle of salt. Do not use foods which contain salt, such as soup, bacon, smoked ham, canned chicken, or fish containing salt, frankfurters, bologna, canned or spiced meat, or salted butter.

Second course of each meal: This part of the diet is strictly limited.

At each meal you have a choice of an ordinary portion of any one of the following: white potatoes, sweet potatoes, boiled rice, half grapefruit, grapes, slice of melon, a banana, a pear, raspberries or blueberries.

At the end of each meal have a cup of black coffee or tea without sugar. Do not use saccharine.

Be sure to drink 6 glasses of water every day before five o'clock. Your only other beverage is half a lemon in a glass of water if you desire it.

This diet contains no bread, flour, salt, sugar, alcohol, or anything else not mentioned.

Treatment of OBESITY with Calorically UNRESTRICTED DIETS. - 1953

The rate of weight loss has been shown to be proportional to the deficiency in calorie intake when the proportions of macronutrients are kept constant, however, the rate of weight loss varies greatly on diets of different composition.

When calorie intake was constant at 1,000 per day, it

was most rapid with high-fat diets; it was less rapid with high-protein diets; and weight could be maintained for short periods on diets of chiefly carbohydrate.

At a level of intake of 2,000 calories per day, weight was maintained or increased in four out of five obese patients unless on the low-carb diet, and significant weight loss still occurred when calorie intake was raised to 2,600 per day, provided this intake was given mainly in the form of fat and protein.

Calorie intake in relation to body-weight changes in the obese. - 1956

5 obese women were fed 400 calories from single energy sources and 800 calorie combinations of these.

Loss of weight was much greater with diets based on fat than on carbohydrate.

Ketosis, weight loss, uric acid, and nitrogen balance in obese women fed single nutrients at low caloric levels - 1969

Moderately obese young college men pursuing their usual activities were studied first during a 3-week prereduction weight maintenance period and subsequently were distributed into 3 isocaloric, isoprotein diet subgroups, which varied as to level of carbohydrate in the diet.

On the 1,800-kcal reduction diet consumed over a 9-week period, diet A contained 104 g carbohydrate/day; diet B, 60 g; diet C, 30 g. The three-man subgroups were matched as closely as possible on the basis of maintenance caloric requirement and percent body weight as fat.

Weight loss, fat loss, and percent weight loss as fat appeared to be inversely related to the level of carbohydrate.

Effect on body composition and other parameters in obese young men of carbohydrate level of reduction diet. - 1971

Obese subjects treated with a high fat (~150g), low carbohydrate diet (~50-60g) demonstrated an average daily weight reduction of 0.3kg/day.

Response of body weight to a low carbohydrate, high fat diet in normal and obese subjects. - 1973

Two isocaloric reducing diets (10cal/kg bodyweight) were studied, one high in fat and low in carbohydrate content, the other high in carbohydrate and low in fat.

The high fat-low carbohydrate diet resulted in a greater weight loss during the 2-week observation period.

Effect of diet composition on metabolic adaptations to hypocaloric nutrition: comparison of high carbohydrate and high fat isocaloric diets. - 1977

In comparative studies, obese patients given a low calorie diet which was low-carbohydrate lost ~14.0kg whilst those given the same calories on a high-carbohydrate diet ~9.8kg. The degree of weight loss was significantly different. Daily weight losses were ~362g and ~298g respectively.

Comparative studies of high and low-carbohydrate formula diets with a greater number of calories did not show any significant difference. However, there was a greater mean weight loss with the low-carbohydrate diet (~351 g/day) compared with that under the high-carbohydrate diet (~296 g/day).

Evaluation of 117 patients treated with formula diets resulted in a weight loss of over ~9kg in 102 obese patients and over ~18 kg in 52 patients. The good response to the low-carbohydrate diet was partly responsible for the successful therapy.

Dietetic treatment of obesity with low and high-carbohydrate diets:
comparative studies and clinical results. - 1979

24 obese but otherwise normal men and women were followed for 2 weeks on their usual food intake; eight weeks on a high-protein, low-carbohydrate diet; and then again for 2 weeks on their usual diet.

The high-protein, low-carbohydrate dieting resulted in substantial weight loss. Plasma triglycerides fell as well.

Effects of high-protein, low-carbohydrate dieting on plasma lipoproteins
and body weight. - 1980

6 moderately obese, untrained subjects were fed a eucaloric, balanced diet for 2 weeks, followed by 6 weeks of a protein-supplemented fast, which provided 1.2g of protein/kg ideal body weight, supplemented with minerals and vitamins.

The mean weight loss was ~10.6kg.

Isocaloric 1,340 kcal diets involving the isocaloric exchange of fat and carbohydrate were fed to obese persons.

The weight loss observed during the carbohydrate-restricted diets was significantly greater than during the high-carbohydrate diet.

After 28 days of treatment the weight loss recorded:

- high-carbohydrate diet: ~9.5kg
- corn oil diet ~11.4kg
- butter diet ~12.5kg

From the findings obtained it appears that the alterations in the water and electrolyte balance observed during the low-carbohydrate diets are reversible phenomena and should thus not be regarded as causal agents of the different weight reduction.

6 adolescents weighing an average of ~148kg were put on an energy restricted diet of ~700 calories, 25g of each fat and carbs, the rest of which derived from protein. A ketogenic regime commonly known as a protein sparing modified fast.

After 8 weeks the subjects lost ~15kg, predominantly fat.

Experiments have shown that the amount and source of dietary energy may alter protein metabolism.

Adult rats were fed diets of either high carb or high fat, final body weight was lower in rats fed the high fat diet, and also had the highest nitrogen balance.

Rats fed the high fat diet had the highest protein gain and the lowest fat gain as a function of energy gain.

Influence of dietary carbohydrate-to-fat ratio on whole body nitrogen retention and body composition in adult rats. - 1989

65 healthy overweight subjects were put on ad libitum low-fat diets for 6 months that were either low or moderate protein, making both diets high carbohydrate but modestly lower in the higher protein version.

Weight loss after 6 months was ~5.1kg in the low protein group and ~8.9 kg in the higher protein group, and fat loss was ~4.3kg and ~7.6kg, respectively.

Replacement of seemingly minor amounts of dietary carbohydrate by protein in an ad libitum fat-reduced diet, improves weight loss and increases the proportion of subjects achieving a clinically relevant weight loss.

Randomized trial on protein vs carbohydrate in ad libitum fat reduced diet for the treatment of obesity. - 1999

24 subjects completed a 12-week high monounsaturated fat, very low carbohydrate programme.

The average weight loss was ~9.1 kg and the average waist measurement was reduced from ~117 to ~105cm.

Metabolic and Anthropometric changes in obese subjects from an unrestricted calorie, high monounsaturated fat, very low carbohydrate diet.
- 2000

A high-carbohydrate, low-fat meal was administered to 6 lean and 7 overweight men after a 17.5-h fast, the overweight group showed a greater energy expenditure, higher protein oxidation, and a lower fat oxidation than did the lean men.

De novo lipogenesis (new fat creation) was significantly higher in the overweight men.

Postprandial de novo lipogenesis and metabolic changes induced by a high-carbohydrate, low-fat meal in lean and overweight men. - 2001

The effects of a 6-week carbohydrate-restricted diet were fat mass was significantly decreased (-3.4 kg) and lean body mass significantly increased (+1.1 kg).

Body composition and hormonal responses to a carbohydrate-restricted diet. - 2002

41 overweight or obese people were placed on a very low carbohydrate diet with no limit on caloric intake for 6

months, mean body weight decreased ~10%.

Effect of 6-month adherence to a very low carbohydrate diet program. -
2002

20 women completed an 8-week trial that reduced their daily carbohydrate intake from ~232g to ~71g without changes in protein or fat consumption.

The average weight loss was ~5.0 kg.

Effects of a hypocaloric, low-carbohydrate diet on weight loss, blood lipids, blood pressure, glucose tolerance, and body composition in free-living overweight women. - 2002

11 obese women were randomly assigned to a 10 week dietary intervention study comparing high protein or high carb energy restricted diets.

On average, the individuals on the high protein dietary group lost ~4.4 kg more than those in the high carb program which was mainly due to a fat mass loss with no statistical differences in lean body mass reduction.

Effects of protein vs. carbohydrate-rich diets on fuel utilisation in obese women during weight loss. - 2003

37 obese children were put on a diet of either ad-libitum very low carb or a low calorie balanced diet for 2 months.

Subjects in the very low carb group lost ~5.2kg whereas the subjects restricting calories actually gained ~2.4kg.

132 severely obese subjects with a high prevalence of diabetes or metabolic syndrome were assigned to a carbohydrate-restricted or a calorie- and fat-restricted diet.

Subjects on the low-carbohydrate diet lost more weight (~5.8kg) than those on the low-fat diet (1.9kg).

A Low-Carbohydrate as Compared with a Low-Fat Diet in Severe Obesity. - 2003

Healthy but obese women were assigned either a very low carbohydrate or a low fat diet for 6 months.

Compared with the low fat group, who followed a diet conforming to currently recommended distributions of macronutrient calories, the very low carbohydrate group lost significantly more weight.

Body composition showed that the weight lost in the very low carbohydrate diet group consisted of a similar percentage of fat mass as in the low fat diet group. Thus, we think it is very unlikely that differences are a result of disproportionate changes in body water in the very low carbohydrate dieters.

The reduction in daily caloric intake was similar in the two groups. For the greater weight loss in the very low carbohydrate group to be strictly a result of decreased caloric consumption, they would have had to consume approximately 300 fewer calories per day over the first 3 months relative to the low fat diet group.

A Randomized Trial Comparing a Very Low Carbohydrate Diet and a Calorie-Restricted Low Fat Diet on Body Weight and Cardiovascular Risk Factors in Healthy Women. - 2003

The study group was instructed to consume <20 g of carbohydrate per day for 2 weeks, then <40 g/day for 10 weeks, and to eat low carbohydrate foods according to hunger. The control group was instructed to consume <30% of energy from fat.

The low carbohydrate group lost more weight, ~9.9kg vs ~4.1kg.

Effects of a low-carbohydrate diet on weight loss and cardiovascular risk factor in overweight adolescents. - 2003

23 obese non-diabetic patients with CVD were put on a high saturated fat and zero starch diet.

After 6 weeks they had lost ~5% total bodyweight, 15 of them with polycystic ovary syndrome after 24 weeks lost ~14%, and eight of them with reactive hypoglycemia after 52 weeks lost ~20% total bodyweight.

Effect of a high saturated fat and no-starch diet on serum lipid subfractions in patients with documented atherosclerotic cardiovascular disease. - 2003

83 obese patients put on a ketogenic diet for 24 weeks, resulting in significant weight loss (~14kg), reduction of total cholesterol, it decreased the level of triglycerides,

LDL cholesterol and blood glucose, and increased the level of HDL cholesterol.

Administering a ketogenic diet for a relatively longer period of time did not produce any significant side effects in the patients. Therefore, the present study confirms that it is safe to use a ketogenic diet for a longer period of time than previously demonstrated.

Long-term effects of a ketogenic diet in obese patients. - 2004

15 overweight men consumed 2 diets for 2 consecutive 6-week periods, a very low-carbohydrate and the other a low-fat diet.

Subjects lost significantly more weight during the very low-carbohydrate diet period (~6.1kg) compared with the low-fat diet period (~3.9kg).

Very Low-Carbohydrate and Low-Fat Diets Affect Fasting Lipids and Postprandial Lipemia Differently in Overweight Men. - 2004

120 overweight subjects assigned either a low carb or low fat diet for 24 weeks.

A greater proportion of the low-carbohydrate diet group than the low-fat diet group completed the study (~76% vs ~57%).

Weight loss was greater in the low-carbohydrate diet group (~12.7kg) than in the low-fat diet group (~7.2kg). Patients in both groups lost substantially more fat mass than fat-free mass.

A Low-Carbohydrate, Ketogenic Diet versus a Low-Fat Diet To Treat

Weight Loss   173

132 obese adults assigned either a low carb or low fat restricted calorie diet for 1 year.

Weight loss was similar between groups (~5.1kg on low carb, ~3.1kg on low fat), but effects on atherogenic dyslipidemia and glycemic control were still more favorable with a low-carbohydrate diet after adjustment for differences in weight loss.

The Effects of Low-Carbohydrate versus Conventional Weight Loss Diets in Severely Obese Adults: One-Year Follow-up of a Randomized Trial. - 2004

60 overweight people were assigned to either the US National Cholesterol Education Program (NCEP) diet or a modified low carb (MLC) diet for 12 weeks.

Weight loss was significantly greater in the MLC (~6.1kg) than in the NCEP group (~3.4kg).

The national cholesterol education program diet vs a diet lower in carbohydrates and higher in protein and monounsaturated fat: A randomized trial. - 2004

Despite having similar mean bodyweight, rats given high-GI food had almost twice the body fat of those on a low-GI diet after 9 weeks.

Effects of dietary glycaemic index on adiposity, glucose homoeostasis, and plasma lipids in animals. - 2004

28 healthy, overweight/obese men and women were prescribed two energy-restricted (-500 kcal/day) diets: a ketogenic diet, and a low fat diet with a goal similar to national recommendations.

Daily calories on the ketogenic diet for the men were ~1,855 compared to the ~1,562 on low fat. A distinct advantage of keto over low fat was demonstrated for weight loss, total fat loss, and trunk fat loss for men.

The majority of women also responded more favorably to the ketogenic diet, especially in terms of trunk fat loss.

Individual responses clearly show the majority of men and women experience greater weight and fat loss on a low carb than a low fat diet.

Comparison of energy-restricted very low-carbohydrate and low-fat diets on weight loss and body composition in overweight men and women. - 2004

96 insulin-resistant women were randomised to one of 3 dietary interventions: a high-carbohydrate, high-fibre (HC) diet, the high-fat (HF) Atkins Diet, or the high-protein (HP) Zone Diet. There were supervised weight loss and weight maintenance phases (8 weeks each).

When compared with the HC diet, the HF and HP diets were shown to produce significantly greater reductions weight loss, waist circumference, and triglycerides.

Comparison of high-fat and high-protein diets with a high-carbohydrate diet in insulin-resistant obese women. - 2005

48 women with BMI >26 were assigned to either a high

carb/moderate protein or moderate carb/high protein diet of 1,700 calories. These groups were then also split into either normal light activity or frequent walking and occasional resistance exercise, averaging ~3.5 hours exercise a week.

All groups lost significant weight during the 16 weeks, the lower carb groups moreso than the high carb groups (~9.3kg vs ~7.3kg).

The exercise treatment did not affect weight loss, however those in the exercise groups lost more fat vs lean than the non-exercise groups.

Dietary protein and exercise have additive effects on body composition during weight loss in adult women. - 2005

11 women with a BMI >27 and a clinical diagnosis of PCOS were instructed to limit their carbohydrate intake to 20 grams or less per day for 24 weeks.

All subjects who participated through 24 weeks lost weight. The overall mean body weight change from baseline to 24 weeks was -12.1%.

The effects of a low-carbohydrate, ketogenic diet on the polycystic ovary syndrome: a pilot study. - 2005

13 overweight women consumed 20g or less carbohydrate/day with liberal intakes of protein and fat for 2 weeks; thereafter, carbohydrate intake increased 5g/week for 10 weeks.

Ketone production was highest at week 1 and declined weekly and was correlated with presence of urinary ketones, but no relationship was found between weekly weight change and serum ketone production.

Urinary ketones reflect serum ketone concentration but do not relate to weight loss in overweight premenopausal women following a low-carbohydrate/high-protein diet. - 2005

13 overweight women consumed a low-carbohydrate/high-protein whilst 15 followed a high-carbohydrate/low-fat diet for 6 weeks.

All women experienced a reduction in bodyweight, although relative loss was greater in the low-carbohydrate/high-protein vs high-carbohydrate/low-fat group.

Perceived Hunger Is Lower and Weight Loss Is Greater in Overweight Premenopausal Women Consuming a Low-Carbohydrate/High-Protein vs High-Carbohydrate/Low-Fat Diet. - 2005

21 overweight participants with type 2 diabetes maintained a ketogenic diet for 16-weeks with an initial goal of <20g/day of carbohydrate.

The mean body weight decreased significantly (~9kg), BMI decreased from ~42 to ~39.

A low-carbohydrate, ketogenic diet to treat type 2 diabetes. - 2005

102 patients with Type 2 diabetes were randomly allocated to a restricted carbohydrate or a reduced-portion, low-fat diet.

Weight loss was greater in the low-carbohydrate group (~3.5kg vs. ~0.9kg).

Short-term effects of severe dietary carbohydrate-restriction advice in Type 2 diabetes—a randomized controlled trial. - 2006

29 overweight men consumed an ad libitum low carb (13%) diet for 12 weeks, weight loss was ~7.5kg.

Effects of a carbohydrate-restricted diet on emerging plasma markers for cardiovascular disease. - 2006

29 overweight men participated in a weight loss intervention diet with a macronutrient energy distribution of ~10% carbohydrate, ~65% fat, and ~25% protein.

After 12 weeks, subjects had a mean weight loss of ~7.5 kg and abdominal fat was reduced by ~20%.

Carbohydrate Restriction Alters Lipoprotein Metabolism by Modifying VLDL, LDL, and HDL Subfraction Distribution and Size in Overweight Men. - 2006

30 patients (15 study subjects and 15 controls) were recruited for this 3-month study. The 15 patients on the diet were instructed to consume less than 20 g of carbohydrates per day for the 1st month and then less than 40 g per day for months 2 and 3. Control subjects had no restrictions on their diet.

The dieters lost ~6.4kg versus ~1kg for the controls at 3 months.

66 healthy obese subjects with BMI >30 were put on a ketogenic diet for 56 weeks.

The body weight and body mass index of all decreased significantly.

Long term effects of ketogenic diet in obese subjects with high cholesterol level. - 2006

Moderately obese subjects consumed two different low carb diets as part of a weight loss regimen:

1) a diet high in foods of mammalian origin intended to contain more saturated fat, or

2) a diet high in poultry, fish, and shellfish, intended to contain more PUFA.

Both diets were associated with significant weight loss after 28 days.

Effects of low carbohydrate diets high in red meats or poultry, fish and shellfish on plasma lipids and weight loss. - 2007

5 patients with a mean BMI of ~36 were instructed to follow a ketogenic diet with nutritional supplementation for 6 months.

The mean weight loss was ~13kg.

The Effect of a Low-Carbohydrate, Ketogenic Diet on Nonalcoholic Fatty

64 obese diabetic subjects on a ketogenic diet for 56 weeks lost significant body weight and saw a significant reduction in BMI.

Beneficial effects of ketogenic diet in obese diabetic subjects. - 2007

311 obese women were assigned one of 4 weight-loss diets representing a spectrum of low to high carbohydrate intake for effects on weight loss and related metabolic variables over 12 months.

Mean 12-month weight loss was as follows:

- Atkins, −4.7 kg
- Zone, −1.6 kg
- LEARN, −2.6 kg
- Ornish, −2.2 kg

Subjects assigned to follow the Atkins diet, which had the lowest carbohydrate intake, lost more weight and experienced more favorable overall metabolic effects than those assigned to follow the Zone, Ornish, or LEARN diets.

Comparison of the atkins, zone, ornish, and learn diets for change in weight and related risk factors among overweight premenopausal women: The a to z weight loss study: a randomized trial. - 2007

Mice were fed one of four diets: a ketogenic diet; an obesegenic diet high in fat and carbohydrate; a calorie restricted diet; and a control diet.

The keto, obesegenic, and control diets were all the same amount of calories.

Mice on keto and calorie restricted both dropped to ~85% of initial weight.

Mice made obese on the high fat/carb diet were then put on keto and lost all excess weight.

A high-fat, ketogenic diet induces a unique metabolic state in mice. - 2007

93 overweight or obese participants were randomly assigned to an energy-restricted isocaloric LCHF diet or an HCLF diet for 8 weeks.

The LCHF diet resulted in significantly greater weight loss than did the HCLF diet.

Low- and high-carbohydrate weight-loss diets have similar effects on mood but not cognitive performance. - 2007

13 diabetic and non-diabetic subjects were each randomly allocated to either a low-carbohydrate diet or a healthy-eating diet following Diabetes UK nutritional recommendations for 3 months.

Weight loss was greater in the low-carbohydrate group (~6.9kg vs ~2.1kg).

A low-carbohydrate diet is more effective in reducing body weight than healthy eating in both diabetic and non-diabetic subjects. - 2007

17 obese men were studied in a residential trial; food was provided daily. Subjects were offered 2 high-protein ad libitum diets, a ketogenic diet and a moderate carb diet.

Ad libitum energy intakes were lower with the ketogenic diet, over the 4 week period weight loss was significantly greater .

Effects of a high-protein ketogenic diet on hunger, appetite, and weight loss in obese men feeding ad libitum. - 2008

99 overweight/obese subjects were put on either a low carb or high carb diet which was calorie restricted by ~30% for 8 weeks.

Weight loss occurred in both groups and was greater in the low carb group (~7.9kg vs ~6.5kg).

Effects of weight loss from a very-low-carbohydrate diet on endothelial function and markers of cardiovascular disease risk in subjects with abdominal obesity. - 2008

55 people of ~33 BMI were put on diets restricted by ~500 calories for 4 months, of either 1.6g/kg protein and <170g carbohydrate, or 0.8g/kg protein and >220g carbohydrate.

There was a trend for lower carb to lose more weight (~9.1% vs ~7.3%) and a higher proportion of fat mass.

Moderate carbohydrate, moderate protein weight loss diet reduces cardiovascular disease risk compared to high carbohydrate, low protein diet in obese adults: A randomized clinical trial. - 2008

31 obese subjects undertook a so-called "Spanish Ketogenic Mediterranean Diet" which is based on fish, green veggies and salads, virgin olive oil, and moderate red wine intake. It is an unlimited calorie diet.

After 3 months the participants had lost ~14kg and reduced their BMI from ~36 to ~31.

Spanish Ketogenic Mediterranean diet: a healthy cardiovascular diet for
weight loss. - 2008

Subjects with type 2 diabetes on a low carbohydrate diet after 6 months had lost ~11kg. In a follow-up after the intervention period at 22 months, mean bodyweight had increased by ~2.7kg, and at 44 months average weight has increased another ~1kg.

Of the 16 patients, five have retained or reduced bodyweight since the 22 month point and all but one have lower weight at 44 months than at start.

Low-carbohydrate diet in type 2 diabetes: stable improvement of
bodyweight and glycemic control during 44 months follow-up. - 2008

Subjects with obesity and type 2 diabetes were randomized to either a low-carbohydrate, ketogenic diet or a low-glycemic, reduced-calorie diet.

The ketogenic group lost ~11.1kg vs. ~6.9 kg lost in the low glycemic participants.

The effect of a low-carbohydrate, ketogenic diet versus a low-glycemic
index diet on glycemic control in type 2 diabetes mellitus. - 2008

In a retrospective review of patients attending an outpatient metabolic management program 31 patients aged ~58 were prescribed a high fat low carb diet.

Subjects lost significant weight even though they were not instructed to reduce energy intake.

Clinical Experience of a Diet Designed to Reduce Aging. - 2009

Subjects were put on a diet restricted by ~500 calories comprised of either 1.6g/kg of protein and <170g of carbohydrates, or 0.8g/kg of protein and >220g of carbs.

After 4 months the protein group had lost slightly more weight (~8.2kg vs ~7kg) and fat mass (~5.6kg vs ~4.6kg). At 12 months the lower carb group had more participants complete the study (64% vs 45%) with greater improvement in body composition, and further weight loss was not significant (~10.4kg vs ~8.4kg).

A moderate-protein diet produces sustained weight loss and long-term changes in body composition and blood lipids in obese adults. - 2009

19 obese men were randomized to a low-fat diet comprised of either normal or increased-protein diet for 8 weeks.

The higher-protein diet produced a greater weight loss, ~8.3% vs ~5.5.

Effects of two energy-restricted diets differing in the carbohydrate/protein ratio on weight loss and oxidative changes of obese men. - 2009

This systematic review included all known randomised controlled trials of low carb vs low fat diets from 2000 to 2007. Factors including weight, cholesterol, blood pressure and glycemic control were evaluated, as these are important in weight loss and cardiovascular disease risk.

Evidence demonstrates that low carb and high protein diets are more effective at 6 months and are as effective, if not more, as low fat diets in reducing weight and cardiovascular disease risk up to 1 year.

Systematic review of randomized controlled trials of low-carbohydrate vs. low-fat/low-calorie diets in the management of obesity and its comorbidities. - 2009

39 participants with metabolic syndrome followed a lowish-carb diet, simply by eliminating rice and bread, reducing yogurt and milk, and consuming only 1 fruit per day to bring carbohydrate down to ~25%.

After 6 weeks body weight decreased ~13%, at which stage 19 were randomly switched to the AHA diet of 55% carbohydrate.

After 12 weeks, body weight was lower in the carb-restricted group than in the subjects who switched to the AHA diet, both groups consumed a similar amount of energy at week 12; thus, energy intake cannot be related to the extent of weight loss difference between groups.

Carbohydrate Restriction, as a First-Line Dietary Intervention, Effectively Reduces Biomarkers of Metabolic Syndrome in Emirati Adults. - 2009

In a 12-week study comparing a low carb to a low fat diet on 40 subjects - despite similar reductions in calories to ~1,500 - weight loss in the carbohydrate restricted group was, on average, twofold greater than in the low-fat group (~10.1 kg vs ~5.2 kg).

Carbohydrate Restriction has a More Favorable Impact on the Metabolic Syndrome than a Low Fat Diet. - 2009

60 obese subjects about ~49 years old were randomly assigned to an energy restricted isocaloric low or high carb diet for 8 weeks.

Weight loss was greater in low carb (~8.4kg) compared with high carb (~6.7kg).

Effects of a low carbohydrate weight loss diet on exercise capacity and tolerance in obese subjects. - 2009

Untrained overweight women were put on either a regular diet or low carb diet, and performed performed 60-100 min of varied resistance exercise twice weekly for 10 weeks.

Subjects on the low carb regime lost ~5.6kg of fat mass with no significant change in lean body mass, while the normal dieters gained ~1.6kg with no significant change in fat mass.

Resistance training in overweight women on a ketogenic diet conserved lean body mass while reducing body fat. - 2010

Severely obese adolescents were randomized to either a low carbohydrate or low fat regimen for 13 weeks, with follow-up at 36 weeks.

Significant reduction in weight and BMI was achieved in both groups during intervention, and was significantly greater for the low carbohydrate group (~13kg vs ~7kg).

Efficacy and Safety of a High Protein, Low Carbohydrate Diet for Weight Loss in Severely Obese Adolescents. - 2010

Weight loss on obese subjects after a year of a restricted low calorie/low fat diet versus a low carbohydrate diet with unlimited fat and protein were similar after 1 and 2 years.

Weight and metabolic outcomes after 2 years on a low-carbohydrate versus low-fat diet: a randomized trial. - 2010

A prospective study was carried out in 14 obese men who were put on a Spanish Ketogenic Mediterranean Diet for 12 weeks.

There was an extremely significant improvement in body weight (from ~110kg to ~96kg), BMI (from ~37 to ~32), and waist circumference (from ~114cm to ~99cm)

The effect of the Spanish Ketogenic Mediterranean Diet on nonalcoholic fatty liver disease: a pilot study - 2011

22 obese subjects with metabolic syndrome followed a Spanish Ketogenic Mediterranean Diet for 12 weeks.

Body weight was reduced by ~15kg, BMI down ~5 points, and waist circumference down ~17cm.

A pilot study of the Spanish Ketogenic Mediterranean Diet: an effective therapy for the metabolic syndrome. 2011

106 subjects were put on a ketogenic diet with unlimited calories.

After 6 weeks there was a significant reduction in BMI and weight, fat mass percentage, and waist circumference.

Effect of ketogenic mediterranean diet with phytoextracts and low carbohydrates/high-protein meals on weight, cardiovascular risk factors, body composition and diet compliance in Italian council employees. - 2011

81 obese women in two cohorts (of 6 and 4 months) were randomized to a low-fat or a low-carbohydrate diet.

Weight loss in both cohorts was more significant in low carb groups (~9kg vs ~5kg).

Adiponectin changes in relation to the macronutrient composition of a weight-loss diet. - 2011

58 obese children were placed on either a ketogenic or low calorie diet for 6 months.

Both groups significantly reduced their weight, fat mass, and waist circumference, but the differences were greater in the ketogenic group.

Metabolic impact of a ketogenic diet compared to a hypocaloric diet in obese children and adolescents. - 2012

In 40 healthy, overweight subjects randomly divided into two groups, both a Mediterranean and ketogenic diet lead to a significant decrease in body weight, however the reduction was significantly greater on keto. The ketogenic diet also lead to increased fat oxidation at rest without any effect on resting energy expenditure.

Medium term effects of a ketogenic diet and a Mediterranean diet on resting energy expenditure and respiratory ratio. - 2012

Reduced resting and total energy expenditure following weight loss is thought to contribute to the prevalence of weight regain after dieting and then resuming a normal diet.

21 overweight young adults were put on a weight loss diet, after achieving 10-15% weight loss they were put on a weight maintenance diet of the same calories, but consisting of either low-fat, low-glycemic index, or very low-carbohydrate. This was done in a controlled 3-way crossover design in random order, each for 4 weeks.

Compared with the pre-weight-loss baseline, the decrease in resting and total energy expenditure was greatest with the low-fat diet, intermediate with the low-glycemic index diet, and least with the very low-carbohydrate diet, meaning the low-fat diet caused as much as a 300 calorie drop in expenditure despite the same intake and activity levels as the low carb diet.

Effects of dietary composition on energy expenditure during weight-loss maintenance. - 2012

In a dynamic time series and structural VAR analyses of U.S. data between 1974 and 2006, and a panel analysis of 164 countries between 2001 and 2010, findings from all analyses suggest that increases in carbohydrates are most strongly and positively associated with increases in obesity prevalence, even when controlling for changes in total caloric intake and occupation-related physical activity.

While increases in consumption of carbohydrates seem to increase overweight prevalence, increases in fat consumption carry the opposite effect.

Macronutrients and Obesity: Revisiting the Calories in, Calories out Framework - 2013

The present meta-analysis aimed to investigate whether individuals assigned to a ketogenic diet achieve better long-term body weight when compared with individuals assigned to a conventional low-fat diet.

Comparison of 1,415 patients demonstrates those assigned to a very-low-carbohydrate ketogenic diet had statistically significant greater weight loss than those assigned to a low fat diet.

Very-low-carbohydrate ketogenic diet v. low-fat diet for long-term weight loss: a meta-analysis of randomised controlled trials. - 2013

Subjects were assigned to either a medium carb/low fat/calorie restricted (MCCR) diet as specified by the American Diabetes Association, or an unrestricted ketogenic diet.

The keto group lost more weight, ~5.5kg vs ~2.6kg.

A Randomized Pilot Trial of a Moderate Carbohydrate Diet Compared to a Very Low Carbohydrate Diet in Overweight or Obese Individuals with Type 2 Diabetes Mellitus or Prediabetes. - 2014

Exercise and Performance

Rates of ketone oxidation and the levels of activity of the enzymes involved in the oxidation of ketones in muscles of exercise-trained and of untrained male rats was measured.

The trained animals had markedly lower blood ketone levels immediately and 60min after a 90min long bout of exercise than did the sedentary animals.

Exercise-induced increase in the capacity of rat skeletal muscle to oxidize ketones. - 1975

Racing sled dogs trained to maximal fitness were put on a zero, lowish, or moderate carbohydrate diet.

No adverse effects were observed in dogs on zero carb, and maintained higher concentrations of albumin, calcium, magnesium, and free fatty acids during the racing season. They also exhibited the greatest increases in red cell count, hemoglobin concentration, and packed cell volume during training.

High values of red cells were not sustained through the racing season in dogs fed the higher carb diet.

The carbohydrate-free, high-fat diet appeared to confer advantages for prolonged strenuous running.

Hematological and metabolic responses to training in racing sled dogs fed diets containing medium, low, or zero carbohydrate. - 1977

To study the capacity for moderate endurance exercise and change in metabolic fuel utilization during adaptation to a ketogenic diet, 6 moderately obese, untrained subjects were fed a eucaloric balanced diet for 2 weeks, followed by 6 weeks of a protein-supplemented fast.

The duration of treadmill exercise to subjective exhaustion was 80% of base line after 1 week of the PSF, but increased to 155% after 6 weeks.

The respiratory quotient (RQ) during steady-state exercise was 0.76 during base line, and fell progressively to 0.66 after 6 weeks of the PSF. Blood glucose was well maintained during exercise in ketosis.

The low RQ and the fact that blood glucose and muscle glycogen were maintained during exhausting exercise after 6 weeks of a PSF suggest that prolonged ketosis results in an adaptation, after which lipid becomes the major metabolic fuel, and net carbohydrate utilization is markedly reduced during moderate but ultimately exhausting exercise.

Capacity for Moderate Exercise in Obese Subjects after Adaptation to a Hypocaloric, Ketogenic Diet. - 1980

5 well-trained cyclists were fed a eucaloric ketogenic diet.

Maximal oxygen uptake (VO2max) was unchanged from baseline after 3 weeks.

Endurance time for continuous exercise to exhaustion at ~63% of VO2max was 147 minutes at baseline and 151 minutes after 4 weeks of keto, with a three-fold drop in glucose oxidation and a four-fold reduction in muscle glycogen use.

These results indicate that aerobic endurance exercise by well-trained cyclists was not compromised by four weeks of ketosis.

The human metabolic response to chronic ketosis without caloric restriction: preservation of submaximal exercise capability with reduced carbohydrate oxidation. - 1983

It is well accepted that exercise endurance is directly related to the amount of carbohydrate stored in muscle and that a low carbohydrate diet reduces glycogen storage and exercise performance. However, more recent evidence has shown that when the organism adapts to a high fat diet endurance is not hindered.

Fat-adapted rats ran as long as carbohydrate-fed animals in spite of lower pre-exercise glycogen levels.

Following 72 hours of recovery on the fat diet, glycogen in muscle had replenished to moderately lower than carbohydrate fed rats, the animals were run to exhaustion a second time and run times were again similar.

When diets were switched after run 1, fat-adapted animals, which received carbohydrates for 72 hours, restored muscle and liver glycogen and then ran longer than CHO-adapted animals that ate fat for 72 hours and that had reduced glycogen repletion.

We conclude that, in contrast to the classic CHO loading studies in humans that involved acute (72 hours) fat feedings and subsequently reduced endurance, rats adapted to a high fat diet do not have a decrease in endurance capacity even after recovery from previous exhausting work bouts.

Rats adapted to a prolonged high fat diet increase maximal O2 uptake and submaximal running endurance.

When training is superimposed to a high fat diet, the most prominent finding is that the diet-induced effects are cumulative with the well-known training effect on VO2max, exercise endurance, oxidative capacity of red muscle, and metabolic responses to exercise, with a further reduction in liver glycogen breakdown.

Additive effects of training and high-fat diet on energy metabolism during exercise - 1991

The effects of 2 weeks of either a high-fat or a high-carbohydrate diet on exercise performance in trained cyclists shows time to exhaustion during high intensity exercise was not significantly different between trials, nor were the rates of muscle glycogen utilization.

Despite a lower muscle glycogen content at the onset of moderate intensity exercise, time to exhaustion was significantly longer after the high fat diet.

Enhanced endurance in trained cyclists during moderate intensity exercise following 2 weeks adaptation to a high fat diet. - 1994

8 healthy untrained men aged ~22 spent 3 days on a control, mixed, or a ketogenic diet of equal energy

content.

In comparison with the normal diet, the ketogenic diet resulted in: increased VO2 max, decreased respiratory exchange ratio an a shift of lactate threshold towards higher exercise loads.

On keto the blood lactate concentrations were lower before, during and after exercise. Post exercise blood pH, as well as pre-and post exercise base excess and bicarbonates were reduced. Resting ketone body concentration was elevated, during a 1h recovery period ketones decreased, while plasma free fatty acids did not change.

Both the pre-and post-exercise levels of adrenaline, noradrenaline, and cortisol were enhanced, whilst plasma insulin concentration was decreased on the ketogenic diet.

The short-term ketogenic diet does not impair aerobic exercise capacity.

Effect of low-carbohydrate-ketogenic diet on metabolic and hormonal responses to graded exercise in men. - 1996

Ketones displace glucose as the predominating fuel for the brain, decreasing the need for glucose synthesis and accordingly spares its precursor, muscle-derived amino acids.

In a rats heart it increased contractility and decreased oxygen consumption.

Ketoacids? Good medicine? - 2003

16 endurance-trained cyclists were assigned randomly to a control group who consumed their habitual or a high fat diet for 15 days.

They performed a 2.5-hour constant-load ride at 70% peak oxygen consumption followed by a simulated 40-km cycling time-trial.

Changes in glucose tolerance and CAT activity were associated with a shift from carbohydrate to fat oxidation during exercise, which occurred within 5 to 10 days of the high fat diet.

During the constant-load ride, the calculated oxidation of muscle glycogen was reduced from 1.5 to 1.0 g/min after 15 days of the high fat diet.

Metabolic adaptations to a high-fat diet in endurance cyclists - 1999

Of 13 male untrained subjects, seven consumed a fat-rich diet and 6 consumed a carbohydrate-rich diet. After 7 weeks of training and diet, 60 min of bicycle exercise was performed at 68% of maximum oxygen uptake.

During exercise, the respiratory exchange ratio was significantly lower in subjects consuming the fat-rich diet. The leg fatty acid uptake and VLDL-triglyceride uptake were both higher in the subjects consuming the fat-rich diet.

Muscle glycogen breakdown was significantly lower in the subjects taking the fat-rich diet.

Fat utilization during exercise: adaptation to a fat-rich diet increases utilization of plasma fatty acids and very low density lipoprotein-triglyceride in humans. - 2001

5 endurance-trained cyclists participated in two 14-day randomized cross-over trials, the high fat diet increased total fat oxidation and reduced total carbohydrate oxidation but did not alter plasma glucose oxidation during exercise.

High fat caused a decreased reliance on muscle glycogen, and improved time trial performance after prolonged exercise.

High-fat diet versus habitual diet prior to carbohydrate loading: effects of exercise metabolism and cycling performance. - 2001

7 cyclists underwent a 2-week adaptation to various diets of difference carbohydrate and fat contents.

The exercise test lasted approximately 5 hours and comprised a 15-minute trial, an incremental test to measure the peak fat-oxidation rate, and a 100-km trial.

The diets had no statistically significant effect on 15-minute performance, in the 100-km time trial, the high-fat and the fat with carbohydrate-loading conditions attenuated the decline in power output observed in the high-carbohydrate condition, power output during the final 5 km of the time trial in the fat with carbo-loading condition was 1.3-fold greater than in the high-carbohydrate condition.

High-fat dietary conditioning increased fat oxidation, and there was some evidence for enhanced ultra-endurance cycling performance relative to high-carbohydrate

Effects of high-fat and high-carbohydrate diets on metabolism and performance in cycling. - 2002

11 duathletes ingested high-fat or high-carbohydrate diets for 5 weeks in a randomized crossover design.

Oxidative capacity in the muscles was not different after the two diet periods. Muscular fat stores significantly increased after high fat compared with high carb. Glycogen content was not significantly lower after high fat compared to carb.

Maximal power during an incremental exercise test to exhaustion, total work output during a 20-min all-out time trial, as well as half-marathon running time were not different between high fat and high carb.

Blood lactate concentrations and respiratory exchange ratios were significantly lower after high fat than high carb at rest and during all submaximal exercise loads.

Effects of dietary fat on muscle substrates, metabolism, and performance in athletes. - 2003

Impaired physical performance is a common but not obligate result of a low carbohydrate diet.

Time for adaptation, optimized sodium and potassium nutriture, and constraint of protein to 15–25% of daily energy expenditure allow unimpaired endurance performance despite nutritional ketosis.

Examining the results of two ketogenic diet performance studies together indicates that both groups experienced a lag in performance across the first week or two of carbohydrate restriction, after which both peak aerobic power and endurance performance were fully restored. In both studies, one with untrained subjects and the other with highly trained athletes who maintained their training throughout the study, there was no loss of VO2max despite the virtual absence of dietary carbohydrate for 4–6 weeks.

None of the comparative low-carbohydrate versus high-carbohydrate studies done in support of the carbohydrate loading hypothesis sustained the low carbohydrate diet for more than 2 weeks.

Ketogenic diets and physical performance. - 2004

Mice made obese on a diet high in both fat and carbohdrate were then put on a ketogenic regimen, lost all excess weight, and spontaneously increased energy expenditure.

A high-fat, ketogenic diet induces a unique metabolic state in mice. - 2007

Ketogenic diets could increase performance in aerobic sports.

Ketogenic diets: additional benefits to the weight loss and unfounded secondary effects - 2008

10 recreationally active women followed low fat high carb diet and a high protein moderate carb diet for a week each in a random counterbalanced design.

Body weight, body fat and respiratory exchange ratio were significantly reduced following the high-protein diet, but no differences were found in any of the strength performance parameters or the responses of heart rate, systolic and diastolic arterial pressure, blood lactate and blood glucose to exercise.

An isoenergetic high-protein, moderate-fat diet does not compromise strength and fatigue during resistance exercise in women. - 2008

60 obese subjects about ~49 years old were randomly assigned to an energy restricted isocaloric low or high carb diet for 8 weeks.

Peak oxygen uptake and heart rate were unchanged in both groups, fat oxidation increased during submaximal exercise in low but not high carb groups.

On both diets, perception of effort during submaximal exercise and handgrip strength decreased, but knee extensor strength remained unchanged.

The low carb diet had no detrimental effect on maximal or submaximal markers of aerobic exercise performance or muscle strength compared with a high carb diet.

Effects of a low carbohydrate weight loss diet on exercise capacity and tolerance in obese subjects. - 2009

8 athletes were analyzed for body composition and various performance aspects before and after 30 days of a modified ketogenic diet. The diet was based on green vegetables, olive oil, fish and meat plus dishes composed of high quality protein and virtually zero carbohydrates.

No significant differences were detected between the ketogenic and standard diet in all strength tests.

Significant differences were found in body weight and body composition: after keto there was a decrease in body weight and fat mass with a non-significant increase in muscle mass.

Ketogenic diet does not affect strength performance in elite artistic gymnasts. - 2012

Subjects with strength training experience performed a variety of tests after a week of a habitual moderate carb diet then again after a week on a very low carb diet.

Body mass decreased significantly, despite this, strength and power outputs were maintained for both men and women.

Effects of a short-term carbohydrate-restricted diet on strength and power performance. - 2013

The Brain, Neurodegenerative Disease, Epilepsy, Cognition, Depression

31% of patients who had idiopathic epilepsy were rendered free of attacks and 16% became definitely improved when the ketogenic diet was given an adequate trial. In all, 47% benefited.

8% whose seizures were controlled by the ketogenic diet had recurrence of attacks within 7 years following the last attack. No recurrence occurred after more than 7 years.

RESULTS OF 15 YEARS' EXPERIENCE WITH THE KETOGENIC DIET IN THE TREATMENT OF EPILEPSY IN CHILDREN. - 1938

A group of obese men with no significant blood ketones injected with insulin suffered clinical signs of hypoglycaemia as their brain became starved of glucose.

After two months of fasting the subjects ketone levels were around ~8.0, in this case the insulin shot dropped the blood glucose levels even further to levels associated with coma and likely death, but they suffered no ill consequences of glucose starvation in the brain as the high ketone levels were more than adequate to fulfill the role.

Resistance to symptomatic insulin reactions after fasting. - 1972

Rats on a high fat diet for 3 weeks had significantly

better concentrations and binding of various compounds in the brain, along with an increase in cerebral energy reserves and charge.

Chronic ketosis and cerebral metabolism. - 1978

When exposed to hypoxia, mice with elevated blood ketones live longer than mice with normal blood ketones.

Reducing available oxygen from 95%, in steps, to 5% produced the expected gradual reduction in the carbon dioxide formation from glucose.

In contrast, reducing the oxygen level to 40 and 20% resulted in a statistically significant stimulation of the production of carbon dioxide from the ketone beta-hydroxybutyrate.

If the increase in carbon dioxide production from ketones can be equated with an increase in energy production from this supplemental substrate then ketones may be therapeutically useful in avoiding the collapse of brain function during moderate hypoxia.

Hypoxia induced preferential ketone utilization by rat brain slices. - 1984

Rats fed a low protein diet which is high in fat retained normal brain glucose utilisation even in a low blood glucose scenario.

However in a low protein and low fat scenario where the fat is swapped out for carbohydrates it results in the rats depressed ability to use glucose in the central nervous system, to a degree seen in brain disorder levels.

29 depressed subjects and a matched group of nondepressed subjects completed a 3-day food record. Results revealed that depressed and nondepressed groups consume similar amounts of all nutrients except protein and carbohydrates.

Nondepressed subjects consume more protein and depressed subjects consume more carbohydrates.

Comparison of nutrient intake among depressed and nondepressed individuals. - 1996

20 healthy volunteers consumed a diet of moderate fat for 1 month, then for the next month half of the subjects changed to a low-fat diet and the remainder continued on moderate fat.

Profile of mood states ratings of anger-hostility significantly increased on the low-fat diet, while there was a slight decline in anger-hostility in the control subjects.

Alterations in mood after changing to a low-fat diet. - 1998

150 children with epilepsy taking at least 2 medications were put on a keto diet.

Approximately ⅓ of the subjects had their seizure rate reduced by over 90% within 3 months.

51 children with intractable seizures were treated with the ketogenic diet.

3 months after initiating the diet, frequency of seizures was decreased to greater than 50% in 54%. At 6 months, 28 of the 51 initiating the diet had at least a 50% decrease from baseline, and at 1 year, 40% of those starting the diet had a greater than 50% decrease in seizures. Five patients were free of seizures at 1 year.

A multicenter study of the efficacy of the ketogenic diet. - 1998

Elevation of ketones may offer neuroprotection in the treatment or prevention of both Alzheimer's disease, where therapy is lacking, and Parkinson's disease, where therapy with L-dopa is time limited.

d-β-Hydroxybutyrate protects neurons in models of Alzheimer's and Parkinson's disease - 2000

A retrospective review of 32 infants who had been treated with the ketogenic diet were able to maintain strong ketosis. The overall effectiveness of the diet in infants was similar to that reported in the literature for older children.

The diet was particularly effective for patients with infantile spasms/myoclonic seizures. There were concomitant reductions in antiepileptic medications. The majority of parents reported improvements in seizure frequency and in their child's behavior and function, particularly with respect to attention/alertness, activity level, and socialization.

The diet generally was well-tolerated, and 96.4% maintained appropriate growth parameters. The ketogenic diet should be considered safe and effective treatment for infants with intractable seizures.

Experience with the ketogenic diet in infants. - 2001

12 of 14 children suffered seizures on a daily basis prior to the ketogenic diet. Mean time to onset of ketosis was 33 hours and to good ketosis, 58 hours.

5 children experienced success with the ketogenic diet, and all of these had their antiepileptic medications either withdrawn or decreased.

Is a fast necessary when initiating the ketogenic diet? - 2002

18 children with autistic behavior were put on a ketogenic diet for 6 months, with continuous administration for 4 weeks, interrupted by 2-week diet-free intervals.

Significant improvement was recorded in two patients, average improvement in eight patients, and minor improvement in eight patients.

Application of a ketogenic diet in children with autistic behavior: pilot study. - 2003

The ketone body DβHB, a crucial alternative source of glucose for brain energy, confers protection against the structural and functional deleterious effects of the parkinsonian toxin MPTP.

DβHB levels may be a straightforward neuroprotective strategy for the treatment of neurodegenerative diseases.

D-β-Hydroxybutyrate rescues mitochondrial respiration and mitigates features of Parkinson disease. - 2003

It is proposed the metabolic management of epilepsy occurs through two main processes. The first involves a reduction in circulating glucose levels. The second involves an elevation in circulating ketone bodies that replaces the lost energy from glucose. This would shift neurotransmitter pools and modulate membrane excitability thus restoring the physiological balance of excitation and inhibition.

Since the metabolism of ketone bodies is thermodynamically more efficient than the metabolism of glucose, a shift in brain energy metabolism from glucose to ketones will produce a homeostatic state that is capable of restoring the physiological balance of excitation and inhibition.

Perspectives on the metabolic management of epilepsy through dietary reduction of glucose and elevation of ketone bodies. - 2003

Ketones displace glucose as the predominating fuel for the brain, decreasing the need for glucose synthesis and accordingly spares its precursor, muscle-derived amino acids.

Without this metabolic adaptation, H. sapiens could not have evolved such a large brain.

Ketones have also protected neuronal cells in tissue culture against exposure to toxins associated with Alzheimer's or Parkinson's in rats.

Ketoacids? Good medicine? - 2003

Normal mammalian brain cells are metabolically versatile and capable of deriving energy from glucose and ketone bodies.

A shift in energy metabolism from glucose to ketones will enhance the bioenergetic potential of normal brain cells.

Role of glucose and ketone bodies in the metabolic control of experimental brain cancer. - 2003

In Alzheimer's disease, there appears to be a pathological decrease in the brain's ability to use glucose. Neurobiological evidence suggests that ketone bodies are an effective alternative energy substrate for the brain.

Elevation of plasma ketone body levels through an oral dose of medium chain triglycerides may improve cognitive functioning in older adults with memory disorders. Higher ketone values were associated with greater improvement in paragraph recall with MCT treatment.

Effects of β-hydroxybutyrate on cognition in memory-impaired adults. - 2004

Individuals with epilepsy often have behavioral problems and deficits in attention and cognitive functioning. The ketogenic diet has been found to effect improvements in these domains. It has also been suggested that the ketogenic diet may act as a mood stabilizer.

In an animal model of depression, rats on the ketogenic diet spent less time immobile, suggesting that rats on the ketogenic diet, like rats treated with antidepressants, are less likely to exhibit "behavioral despair."

The ketogenic diet may have antidepressant properties.

The antidepressant properties of the ketogenic diet. - 2004

The pattern of protection of the ketogenic diet in animal models of seizures is distinct from that of other anticonvulsants, suggesting that it has a unique mechanism of action. During consumption of the ketogenic diet, marked alterations in brain energy metabolism occur, with ketone bodies partly replacing glucose as fuel.

In addition to acute seizure protection, the ketogenic diet has neuroprotective properties in diverse models of neurodegenerative disease.

The Neuropharmacology of the Ketogenic Diet. - 2007

Dietary protocols that increase serum levels of ketones, such as calorie restriction and the ketogenic diet, offer robust protection against a multitude of acute and chronic neurological diseases. The underlying mechanisms, however, remain unclear.

A combination of β-hydroxybutyrate and acetoacetate decreased neuronal death and prevented changes in neuronal membrane properties induced by 10 μM glutamate. Ketones also significantly decreased mitochondrial production of reactive oxygen species and the associated excitotoxic changes by increasing NADH oxidation in the mitochondrial respiratory chain, but did not affect levels of the endogenous antioxidant glutathione.

It is demonstrated that ketones reduce glutamate-induced free radical formation by increasing the NAD+/NADH ratio and enhancing mitochondrial respiration in neocortical neurons. This mechanism may, in part, contribute to the neuroprotective activity of ketones by restoring normal bioenergetic function in the face of oxidative stress.

KETONES INHIBIT MITOCHONDRIAL PRODUCTION OF REACTIVE OXYGEN SPECIES PRODUCTION FOLLOWING GLUTAMATE EXCITOTOXICITY BY INCREASING NADH OXIDATION. - 2007

20 children with intractable epilepsy were randomized to either 10 or 20g of carbohydrates per day for the initial 3 months of a modified Atkins diet, and then crossed over to the opposite amount.

A significantly higher likelihood of seizure reduction was noted for children started on 10g of carbohydrate per day at 3 months.

Most parents reported no change in seizure frequency or ketosis between groups, but improved tolerability with 20g per day.

A randomized, crossover comparison of daily carbohydrate limits using the modified Atkins diet. - 2007

In a comparison of the effects of a low-carbohydrate high-fat diet with a conventional high-carbohydrate low-fat diet on mood and cognitive function, there was evidence for a smaller improvement in cognitive functioning with the low carb diet with respect to speed of processing.

Low- and high-carbohydrate weight-loss diets have similar effects on mood but not cognitive performance. - 2007

Fasting animals after a moderate brain injury resulted in a significant increase in tissue sparing. This 24-hr fast also decreased biomarkers of oxidative stress and calcium loading and increased mitochondrial oxidative phosphorylation in mitochondria isolated from the site of injury.

Insulin administration, designed to mimic the hypoglycemic effect, induced increased mortality, however the administration of ketones resulted in increased tissue sparing.

Fasting is neuroprotective following traumatic brain injury. - 2008

Ketone bodies demonstrate a scavenging capacity for diverse reactive oxygen species, reducing cell death and reactive oxygen species production, prevention of neuronal ATP decline, and prevention of the hypoglycemia-induced increase in lipid peroxidation in the rat hippocampus.

Antioxidant capacity contributes to protection of ketone bodies against oxidative damage induced during hypoglycemic conditions. - 2008

An early feature of Alzheimer's disease is region-specific declines in brain glucose metabolism. Inhibition of glucose metabolism can have profound effects on brain function.

One promising approach is to supplement the normal glucose supply of the brain with ketone bodies. Much of the benefit of ketone bodies can be attributed to their ability to increase mitochondrial efficiency and supplement the brain's normal reliance on glucose.

Ketone bodies as a therapeutic for Alzheimer's disease. - 2008

To determine whether the ketogenic diet improves mitochondrial redox status, adolescent rats were fed a ketogenic or control diet for 3 weeks.

Ketogenic rats showed:

- a twofold increase in GSH and GSH/GSSG ratios (mitochondrial antioxidant)
- increased GCL activity
- up-regulated protein levels of GCL subunitsv
- reduced CoA (indicator of mitochondrial redox status)
- increased lipoic acid (thiol antioxidant)

Together, the results demonstrate that the ketogenic diet up-regulates GSH biosynthesis, enhances mitochondrial antioxidant status, and protects mtDNA from oxidant-induced damage.

The ketogenic diet increases mitochondrial glutathione levels - 2008

Lower ketogenic ratios are frequently as effective as higher ones at controlling seizures, and result in fewer adverse effects. However, a minority of patients experience improved seizure control at higher ratios.

There is evidence, both from studies on the traditional and the modified Atkins diet to suggest that starting at higher ratios may result in better control, but that ratios can often be weaned over time without deterioration of efficacy.

In animals, calorie restriction has an independent anticonvulsant effect, above simply increasing ketosis. In children, the need for calorie restriction is less clear. While avoidance of too many calories may improve efficacy, restriction to 75% of daily requirements is probably excessive.

Ketogenic ratio, calories, and fluids: do they matter? - 2008

The modified Atkins diet (MAD) was created at Johns Hopkins Hospital as an attempt to create a more palatable and less restrictive dietary treatment primarily for children with behavioral difficulties and adolescents that parents and neurologists were reluctant to start on the traditional ketogenic diet.

The MAD was designed to mimic ketosis while providing similar but unlimited quantities of high fat and protein foods, and has been reported as efficacious as a traditional ketogenic diet in eight publications to date by centers in four countries.

The diet is "modified" from the Atkins diet as the "induction phase" of the diet limiting carbohydrates is maintained indefinitely, fat is encouraged (not just allowed), and weight loss is not the goal (unless nutritionally indicated).

There have been 100 reported children and adults started on the diet, 45% have had 50–90% seizure reduction, and 28% >90% seizure reduction.

The Modified Atkins Diet. - 2008

A characteristic of Alzheimer's disease is regional hypometabolism in the brain. This decline in cerebral glucose metabolism occurs before pathology and symptoms manifest, continues as symptoms progress, and is more severe than that of normal aging.

Ketone bodies are an efficient alternative fuel for cells that are unable to metabolize glucose or are 'starved' of glucose.

Hypometabolism as a therapeutic target in Alzheimer's disease. - 2008

This case study follows a 70 year old woman diagnosed with schizophrenia, paranoia, disorganized speech, and hallucinations, including seeing skeletons and hearing voices that told her to hurt herself, since childhood.

A typical day's diet was egg and cheese sandwiches, diet soda, water, pimento cheese, barbequed pork, chicken salad, hamburger helper, macaroni and cheese, and potatoes.

She was put on a ketogenic diet of <20g carbs a day, consisting of unlimited meats and eggs, 4 ounces of hard cheese, 2 cups of salad vegetables, and 1 cup of low-carbohydrate vegetables per day.

After just over a week she was no longer hearing voices or seeing skeletons, there was no change in medication.

After 12 months she had no recurrence of hallucinations, had lost ~10kg, and experienced improvements in energy level.

Even with 2–3 isolated episodes of dietary non-compliance that lasted several days where she ate pasta, bread, and cakes, there was no recurrence of hallucinations.

Schizophrenia, gluten, and low-carbohydrate, ketogenic diets: a case report and review of the literature. - 2009

An expanding body of evidence indicates that ketone bodies are indeed neuroprotective.

Ketone bodies protect neurons against multiple types of neuronal injury and the underlying mechanisms are similar to those of calorie restriction and of the ketogenic diet.

THE NEUROPROTECTIVE PROPERTIES OF CALORIE RESTRICTION, THE KETOGENIC DIET, AND KETONE BODIES. - 2009

Animals with traumatic brain injury were fed either a normal or ketogenic diet.

The results show that brain edema, cytochrome c release, and cellular apoptosis were induced after traumatic brain injury and that a ketogenic diet reduced these changes dramatically.

Ketogenic diet reduces cytochrome c release and cellular apoptosis following traumatic brain injury in juvenile rats - 2009

Aging is associated with increased susceptibility to hypoxic/ischemic insult and declines in behavioral function which may be due to attenuated adaptive/defense responses.

In the aged rats, the ketogenic diet improved cognitive performance under normoxic and hypoxic conditions.

Diet-induced ketosis improves cognitive performance in aged rats. - 2010

Mitochondrial dysfunction is a major cause of neurodegenerative and neuromuscular diseases of adult age and of multisystem disorders of childhood. However, no effective treatment exists for these progressive disorders.

Mice which are a disease model for progressive late-onset mitochondrial myopathy were put on a ketogenic diet, the effects being a decrease in the amount of cytochrome c oxidase negative muscle fibers, a key feature in mitochondrial RC deficiencies, and prevented completely the formation of the mitochondrial ultrastructural abnormalities in the muscle.

Furthermore, most of the metabolic and lipidomic changes were cured by the diet. The diet did not, however, significantly affect the mtDNA quality or quantity, but rather induced mitochondrial biogenesis and restored liver lipid levels.

Ketogenic diet slows down mitochondrial myopathy progression in mice. - 2010

The ketogenic diet has well-established short- and long-term outcomes for children with intractable epilepsy, but only for those actively receiving it.

Of 101 epilepsy patients, with a median current age of 13 years (range 2–26 years) having since discontinued the ketogenic diet (~6 years, range 0.8–14 years), 79% were now similarly improved, 96% would recommend the ketogenic diet to others (only 54% would have started it before trying anticonvulsants).

This is the first study to report on the long-term effects of the ketogenic diet after discontinuation. The majority of subjects are currently doing well with regard to health and seizure control.

Long-term outcomes of children treated with the ketogenic diet in the past.

- 2010

The main clinical symptom of Parkinson's Disease is motor dysfunction derived from the loss of dopaminergic neurons in the substantia nigra and dopamine content in the striatum subsequently. It is well known that treatments with 1-methyl-4-phenyl-1,2,3,6-tetrahydropyridine (MPTP) in mice produce motor dysfunction, biochemical, and neurochemical changes remarkably similar to idiopathic Parkinson's patients.

Pre-treatment with a ketogenic diet alleviated the motor dysfunction induced by MPTP, the decrease of compromised neurons induced by MPTP was inhibited, and the activation of microglia was inhibited.

Neuroprotective and Anti-inflammatory Activities of Ketogenic Diet on MPTP-induced Neurotoxicity. - 2010

Rats which were fasted for 48 hours or following a ketogenic diet increased their ketone and glucose uptake more than 2-fold.

This approach may be particularly interesting in neurodegenerative pathologies such as Alzheimer's disease where brain energy supply appears to decline critically.

Mild experimental ketosis increases brain uptake of 11C-acetoacetate and 18F-fluorodeoxyglucose: a dual-tracer PET imaging study in rats. - 2011

Transgenic Huntington's mice were fed a ketogenic diet ad libitum. There were no usual Huntington's negative effects on any behavioral parameter tested and no significant change in lifespan. Progressive weight loss is a hallmark feature of Huntington's disease, yet the ketogenic diet delayed the reduction in body weight of the transgenic mice.

A ketogenic diet delays weight loss and does not impair working memory or motor function in the R6/2 1J mouse model of Huntington's disease. - 2011

2 year old rats were fed a ketogenic diet for 2 weeks, cerebral metabolic rates of ketones and glucose increased significantly.

The ketogenic diet increases brain glucose and ketone uptake in aged rats: a dual tracer PET and volumetric MRI study. - 2012

The ketogenic diet has a wide range of neurological effects, the following are just some of the spectrum of observations of ketone bodies thus far which require further research:

- raise ATP levels and reduce ROS production, demonstrating neuroprotective properties
- stimulate mitochondrial biogenesis
- stabilise synaptic function
- reduces glycolysis, which suppresses seizures and prolongs lifespan of numerous species
- aged rats have significantly increased mitochondrial density and cerebral function, problem solving and recognition performance
- protect against the toxic effects of ß-amyloid on neurons in culture
- mice benefit from better mitochondrial function, less oxidative stress, and reduced expression of amyloid precursor protein and ß-amyloid
- mitochondrial respiratory chain damage from a toxin is ameliorated in mice
- animals with brain tumors exhibit markedly decreased tumor growth rates
- reductions in ROS production in malignant glioma cells
- rats with induced cardiac arrest and stroke found significantly reduced neurodegeneration
- cognitive and motor functioning are improved
- tissue sparing in brain following injury
- autistic children demonstrate moderate or significant behavioral improvement
- significant reduction in the velocity of cortical spreading depression velocity in immature rats

The ketogenic diet as a treatment paradigm for diverse neurological disorders. - 2012

Central nervous system oxygen toxicity seizures occur with little or no warning, and no effective mitigation strategy has been identified.

Rats were administered a single oral dose of ketone esters to increase ketone body production, then placed into a hyperbaric chamber and pressurized to 5 atmospheres.

Latency to seizure was increased ~574%, the control subjects suffering siezures within ~11 minutes, the ketogenic rats taking almost an hour to capitulate such a fate.

Therapeutic ketosis with ketone ester delays central nervous system oxygen toxicity seizures in rats. - 2013

Bipolar disorder is frequently difficult to treat, and multiple medications are usually required.

Two women with type II bipolar disorder were able to maintain ketosis for prolonged periods of time (2 and 3 years, respectively). Both experienced mood stabilization that exceeded that achieved with medication; experienced a significant subjective improvement that was distinctly related to ketosis; and tolerated the diet well. There were no significant adverse effects in either case.

One reported her diet as diverse with meats (organic grass fed beef, organic pork, and free-range chickens), dairy products (raw whole milk, cream, cheeses), and seafood (salt water fish, clams, shrimp).

The other commented "I find the diet very palatable, and easy to follow. I eat a lot of fish (sardines, salmon, tuna), olive oil, coconut milk, butter, fatty meat, eggs, some bacon, poultry with skin, and some nuts. I use 1–2 tablespoons of coconut oil if I happen to have a few more carbs on any particular day, as this keeps me ketogenic. I have about 1–2 cups of veggies as my daily carb source."

At minimum, these patients' experience suggests that a ketogenic diet, diligently pursued, can act as a mood stabilizer in patients with type II bipolar disorder.

The ketogenic diet for type II bipolar disorder. - 2013

Migraine prophylaxys is an important clinical challenge, sometime complicated by side effects. Among that weight increase is one of most frequent.

Migraine sufferers were assigned either a standard or ketogenic diet, after one month headache frequency and drug consumption was reduced during, but only in the keto group. Responder rates were higher than 90% in terms of attack frequency and drug consumption.

Short term improvement of migraine headaches during ketogenic diet: a prospective observational study in a dietician clinical setting. - 2013

In young adult rats fed 3 weeks of either standard or ketogenic diets, cerebral metabolic rates of glucose significantly decreased in the cerebral cortex and cerebellum with increased plasma ketone bodies in the ketotic rats compared with standard diet group.

Ketosis proportionately spares glucose utilization in brain. - 2013

Juvenile mice with behavioural analogies to autism were fed a ketogenic diet for 3 weeks and tested for sociability, self-directed repetitive behavior, and communication.

They showed increased sociability, decreased self-directed repetitive behavior, and improved social communication of a food preference.

Ketogenic diet improves core symptoms of autism in BTBR mice. - 2013

55 bipolar disorder patients who were non-diabetic, nonpregnant, and drug naïve for a period of at least 6 months demonstrated significantly higher mean levels of fasting plasma insulin, postprandial plasma insulin and a higher value of HOMA-IR.

A significantly higher proportion of bipolar patients compared to controls were manifesting levels of fasting plasma glucose, serum triglyceride and blood pressure higher than the cut off while waist circumference and serum HDL cholesterol failed to show any significant difference in the proportion.

There was a significantly higher proportion of prevalence of insulin resistance between bipolar cases and controls while there was no significant difference in proportion of prevalence of metabolic syndrome between these two groups.

Assessment of insulin resistance and metabolic syndrome in drug naive patients of bipolar disorder. - 2014

Hunger and Appetite Regulation

Any of the low carbohydrate levels [104g / 60g / 30g] in the reduction diet under study were effective in controlling hunger.

Effect on body composition and other parameters in obese young men of carbohydrate level of reduction diet. - 1971

8 women were restricted to 80g of carbohydrate a day but protein and fat were allowed freely.

Energy intake was found to be ~30% lower on this diet than on the subject's habitual diet, but the nutrient content was not reduced.

The Absence of Undesirable Changes during Consumption of the Low Carbohydrate Diet. - 1974

Subjects were fed either a high carbohydrate, high fat, or high protein meal.

The carbohydrate and protein meals increased insulin levels significantly, however not with the fat meal.

The protein meal was also followed by an increase in glucagon, whereas the carbohydrate meal reduced it significantly.

Early insulin and glucagon responses to different food items. - 1996

24 women with BMI >26 were assigned to either a high carb/moderate protein or moderate carb/high protein diet of 1,700 calories, with ~50g coming from fat in each, therefore only modulating the protein and carbohydrate loads.

The high carb diet followed the USDA Food Pyramid which emphasizes the use of breads, rice, cereals and pasta. The high protein diet substituted foods that emphasized animal proteins including red meats, milk, cheese and eggs, with a requirement for a minimum of seven beef meals each week.

Women in the high carb group had higher insulin responses to meals and postprandial hypoglycemia, whereas the high protein dieters reported greater satiety.

A reduced ratio of dietary carbohydrate to protein improves body composition and blood lipid profiles during weight loss in adult women. - 2003

An observation of a randomised controlled trial between an energy unrestricted low carb vs energy restricted low fat diet was the spontaneous reduction of food intake in the low carb group, to a level equal to that of the control subjects who were following a prescribed restriction of calories. This raises the possibility that the very low carbohydrate diet may have been more satiating.

A Randomized Trial Comparing a Very Low Carbohydrate Diet and a Calorie-Restricted Low Fat Diet on Body Weight and Cardiovascular Risk Factors in Healthy Women. - 2003

20 healthy adults were randomly assigned to low-fat

energy-restricted diets of either high-protein or high-carbohydrate.

Subjects consuming the high-protein diet reported more satisfaction and less hunger in month 1 of the trial, and consumed 12–40% less energy in the subsequent 2–3 hours when food was freely available.

Cognitive feelings of less hunger and greater satiety were noted in subjects ingesting high-protein foods, and 2 subjects in the high-carbohydrate group withdrew from the trial due to unendurable hunger.

High-Protein, Low-Fat Diets Are Effective for Weight Loss and Favorably Alter Biomarkers in Healthy Adults. - 2004

10 obese patients with type 2 diabetes followed a low-carbohydrate diet for 14 days, intake was reduced to ~21g/d, but patients could eat as much protein and fat as they wanted and as often as they wanted.

The final diet contained an average of 151g protein, and 164g fat, representing a spontaneous reduction in caloric intake of ~947 calories, from ~3,111 to ~2,164, which resulted in a mean weight loss of ~2kg over 14 days.

Effect of a low-carbohydrate diet on appetite, blood glucose levels, and insulin resistance in obese patients with type 2 diabetes. - 2005

13 overweight women consumed a low-carbohydrate/high-protein whilst 15 followed a high-carbohydrate/low-fat diet for 6 weeks.

Self-rated hunger decreased in women in the low-carbohydrate/high-protein but not in the high-carbohydrate/low-fat group.

Perceived Hunger Is Lower and Weight Loss Is Greater in Overweight Premenopausal Women Consuming a Low-Carbohydrate/High-Protein vs High-Carbohydrate/Low-Fat Diet. - 2005

Following an overnight fast, subjects consumed either an egg or bagel-based breakfast followed by lunch 3.5h later.

During the pre-lunch period, participants had greater feelings of satiety after the egg breakfast, and consumed significantly less energy from all macronutrients for lunch.

Energy intake following the egg breakfast remained lower for the entire day as well as for the next 36 hours.

Short-term effect of eggs on satiety in overweight and obese subjects. - 2005

29 overweight men consumed an ad libitum low carb diet for 12 weeks, energy intake was spontaneously reduced by ~30%.

Effects of a carbohydrate-restricted diet on emerging plasma markers for cardiovascular disease. - 2006

An analysis of the pattern of food consumption during the more recent obesity and diabetes epidemic found that the increase in calories was almost entirely due to an increase in carbohydrate.

Recent research has determined that the reduction in calorie intake is a result of appetite and hunger reduction. In this way, low carb diets are also low-calorie diets that include an increase in the percentage of calories from fat and protein but not necessarily an increase in absolute amounts of fat and protein.

It may also be that the mere lowering of serum insulin concentrations, as is seen with low carb, may lead to a reduction in appetite.

Low-carbohydrate nutrition and metabolism. - 2007

Mood and other symptoms were evaluated by 119 overweight participants self-reporting whilst undergoing weight loss following either a ketogenic diet or a low-fat diet.

Symptoms of hunger improved to a greater degree in patients following a ketogenic diet compared with those following a low fat diet

The effects of a low-carbohydrate ketogenic diet and a low-fat diet on mood, hunger, and other self-reported symptoms. - 2007

17 obese men were studied in a residential trial; food was provided daily. Subjects were offered 2 high-protein ad libitum diets, a ketogenic diet and a moderate carb diet.

Ad libitum energy intakes were lower with the ketogenic diet, over the 4 week period, hunger was significantly lower.

In the short term, high-protein, low-carbohydrate

ketogenic diets reduce hunger and lower food intake significantly more than do high-protein, medium-carbohydrate nonketogenic diets.

Effects of a high-protein ketogenic diet on hunger, appetite, and weight loss in obese men feeding ad libitum. - 2008

Satiety and energy expenditure are important in protein-enhanced weight loss and weight maintenance. Protein-induced satiety has been shown acutely, with single meals, with contents of 25% to 81% of energy from protein in general or from specific proteins, while subsequent energy intake reduction was significant. Protein-induced satiety has been shown with high protein ad libitum diets, lasting from 1 to 6 days, up to 6 months.

Protein-induced satiety: effects and mechanisms of different proteins. - 2008

Ghrelin and peptide YY (PYY) are two hormones produced by the gastrointestinal tract that have effects on appetite. 7-11 year old children were fed a meal either high in fat, carbs, or protein.

After the high-protein meal, ghrelin declined gradually in both groups over the study period without subsequent increase, whereas ghrelin suppressed more rapidly 60 min after the high-carbohydrate meal, followed by rebound in ghrelin levels.

Similarly, after the high-protein meal, PYY concentrations increased steadily over the course of the morning in both groups without decline, whereas PYY levels peaked 30 min after the high-carbohydrate meal with significant decline thereafter.

Ghrelin and PYY responses to the high-fat meal were somewhat intermediate between that observed with high carbohydrate and high protein.

Obese children reported higher hunger and lower satiety after the high-carbohydrate meal compared to the normal weight children subjects, whereas appetite ratings were similar between the groups after the high-protein and high-fat meals.

Effects of meals high in carbohydrate, protein, and fat on ghrelin and peptide YY secretion in prepubertal children. - 2009

Adult rats were divided into 3 groups: normal diet, keto, and high-carbohydrate diet. Diabetes was induced by injection.

Food and water intake were increased in all groups except the keto group.

Therapeutic role of low-carbohydrate ketogenic diet in diabetes. - 2009

This study examined the effects of an eight-week ketogenic diet rich in n-3 fatty acids.

Compared to the habitual diet, subjects consumed significantly greater quantities of protein, fat, MUFA and n-3 fatty acids and significantly less total energy, carbohydrate and dietary fiber.

Fasting lipoprotein and postprandial triglyceride responses to a low-carbohydrate diet supplemented with n-3 fatty acids. - 2000

Exchanging carbohydrate for protein results in increased satiety in women.

Sex differences in energy homeostatis following a diet relatively high in protein exchanged with carbohydrate, assessed in a respiration chamber in humans. - 2009

Appetite suppression and fat oxidation were higher on a high-protein diet with carbohydrates exchanged for fat. Energy expenditure was not affected by the carbohydrate content of a high-protein diet.

Presence or absence of carbohydrates and the proportion of fat in a high-protein diet affect appetite suppression but not energy expenditure in normal-weight human subjects fed in energy balance. - 2010

Obese adults were randomly assigned to a low carb or low fat diet for 2 years. Cravings for specific types of foods (sweets, high-fats, fast-food fats, and carbohydrates/starches); preferences for high-sugar, high-carbohydrate, and low-carbohydrate/high-protein foods; and appetite were measured.

The low carb diet had significantly larger decreases in cravings for carbohydrates/starches and high-sugar foods, and reported being less bothered by hunger, and that men had larger reductions in appetite compared to women.

Change in food cravings, food preferences, and appetite during a low-carbohydrate and low-fat diet. - 2011

22 healthy subjects received a ketogenic zero carb diet or 55% carbohydrate diet of equal calories in a randomised cross-over design.

During the zero carb diet appetite was suppressed.

Gluconeogenesis and protein-induced satiety. - 2012

The circulating concentrations of several hormones and nutrients which influence appetite were altered after weight loss induced by a ketogenic diet, compared with after refeeding. The increase in circulating ghrelin and subjective appetite which accompany dietary weight reduction were mitigated when weight-reduced participants were ketotic.

Ketosis and appetite-mediating nutrients and hormones after weight loss. - 2013

64 participants underwent a meal test of either high carbohydrate/low fat or moderate carb/fat.

The lower carb meal resulted in a later time at the highest and lowest recorded glucose, lower insulin, and reported a lower appetite 3 and 4 hours following the meal.

Modest increases in meal carbohydrate content at the expense of fat content may facilitate weight gain over the long-term by contributing to an earlier rise and fall of postprandial glucose concentrations and an earlier return of appetite.

Return of hunger following a relatively high carbohydrate breakfast is associated with earlier recorded glucose peak and nadir. - 2014

Muscles, Bones, and Body Composition

8 women were restricted to 80g of carbohydrate a day but protein and fat were allowed freely.

During the 6 weeks of the dietary period, the urinary excretion of nitrogen and creatinine were unchanged, indicating no significant loss of tissue protein.

The Absence of Undesirable Changes during Consumption of the Low Carbohydrate Diet. - 1974

Protein intake of 1g/kg vs 2g/kg with either a low, normal or high calcium intake was studied.

During the high protein low and normal calcium intake urinary calcium did not significantly increase. It increased moderately in the higher calcium intakes, however with time they returned to control levels.

Effect of a high protein (meat) intake on calcium metabolism in man. - 1978

During a ketogenic regimen levels of gluconeogenic amino acids are reduced while those of the branched chain amino acids increase.

Hormonal and metabolic changes induced by an isocaloric isoproteinic ketogenic diet in healthy subjects. - 1982

The effect of a high meat diet on calcium metabolism was studied for 78 to 132 days in four adult males and the short-term effect for 18 to 30 days in 3 subjects.

During both studies there was no significant change of the urinary or fecal calcium nor of the calcium balance. There was also no significant change of the intestinal absorption of calcium.

Further studies of the effect of a high protein diet as meat on calcium metabolism. 1983

Adult rats were fed diets of either high carb or high fat, final body weight was lower in rats fed the high fat diet, and also had the highest protein gain.

Influence of dietary carbohydrate-to-fat ratio on whole body nitrogen retention and body composition in adult rats. - 1989

11 out of 20 trauma patients received ketone bodies for 3 hours, resulting in significantly decreased alanine release from muscle suggesting a suppressive effect of ketone bodies on posttraumatic protein catabolism.

Effect of 3-hydroxybutyrate on posttraumatic metabolism in man. - 1991

25 normal glucose-tolerant obese women were put on a low fat 800 calorie diet of either high protein or high carbohydrate for 3 weeks.

Both diets induced a similar decrease in body weight, however excretion of muscle breakdown indicators was reduced by ~48% after the high protein diet.

Hypocaloric high-protein diet improves glucose oxidation and spares lean body mass: comparison to hypocaloric high-carbohydrate diet. - 1994

6 adolescents weighing an average of ~148kg were put on an energy restricted diet of ~700 calories, predominantly protein, a ketogenic regime commonly known as a protein sparing modified fast.

After 8 weeks the subjects lost ~15kg, lean body mass was not significantly affected.

The effects of a high-protein, low-fat, ketogenic diet on adolescents with morbid obesity: body composition, blood chemistries, and sleep abnormalities. - 1998

12 healthy normal-weight men switched from their habitual diet to a carbohydrate-restricted diet for 6 weeks, fat mass was significantly decreased and lean body mass significantly increased.

Body composition and hormonal responses to a carbohydrate-restricted diet. - 2002

A positive association between animal protein consumption and bone mineral density was found to be statistically significant in elderly women.

For every 15g/day increase in animal protein intake, bone mineral density increased.

11 obese women were randomly assigned to a 10 week dietary intervention study comparing high protein or high carb energy restricted diets.

On average, the individuals on the high protein dietary group lost ~4.4kg more than those in the high carb program which was mainly due to a fat mass loss with no statistical differences in lean body mass reduction.

24 women with BMI >26 were assigned to either a high carb/moderate protein or moderate carb/high protein diet of 1,700 calories, with ~50g coming from fat in each, therefore only modulating the protein and carbohydrate loads.

The high carb diet followed the USDA Food Pyramid which emphasizes the use of breads, rice, cereals and pasta. The high protein diet substituted foods that emphasized animal proteins including red meats, milk, cheese and eggs, with a requirement for a minimum of seven beef meals each week.

After 10 weeks both groups lost similar amounts of bodyweight (~7.25kg), but the high protein group was partitioned to a significantly higher loss of fat vs lean than in the high carb group (~6.3kg vs ~3.8kg).

A parallel design included either a high-protein diet of meat, poultry, and dairy foods, or a standard-protein diet low in those foods during 12 weeks of energy restriction and 4 weeks of energy balance.

In women, total lean mass was significantly better preserved with the high protein diet, markers of bone turnover and calcium excretion were unchanged.

Effect of a high-protein, energy-restricted diet on body composition, glycemic control, and lipid concentrations in overweight and obese hyperinsulinemic men and women. - 2003

Ketones displace glucose as the predominating fuel for the brain, decreasing the need for glucose synthesis and accordingly spares its precursor, muscle-derived amino acids.

In a rats heart it increased contractility and decreased oxygen consumption.

Ketoacids? Good medicine? - 2003

Healthy adults were randomly assigned to a low-fat energy-restricted diet of either high-protein or high-carbohydrate, both diets were equally effective at reducing body weight but nitrogen balance was more positive in subjects consuming the high-protein diet.

48 women with BMI >26 were assigned to either a high carb/moderate protein or moderate carb/high protein diet of 1,700 calories. These groups were then also split into either normal light activity or frequent walking and occasional resistance exercise, averaging ~3.5 hours exercise a week.

The high carb diet followed the USDA Food Pyramid which emphasizes restricting fat/cholesterol and the use of breads, rice, cereals and pasta. The high protein diet substituted meats, dairy, and eggs.

All groups lost significant weight, exercise did not affect overall weight loss, however it did preserve significantly more lean mass than the non-exercise groups.

Dietary protein and exercise have additive effects on body composition
during weight loss in adult women. - 2005

Subjects ate a typical Western diet for 2 days, followed immediately by 7 days of a low carb high protein diet.

Muscle protein synthesis and whole-body proteolysis were stimulated without a measurable change in fat free mass.

Effects of Dietary Carbohydrate Restriction with High Protein Intake on
Protein Metabolism and the Somatotropic Axis. - 2005

In a meta-regression analysis of 87 interventional studies, low-carbohydrate, high-protein diets favorably affect body mass and composition independent of energy intake.

Effects of variation in protein and carbohydrate intake on body mass and composition during energy restriction: a meta-regression. - 2006

Low blood sugar is a potent stimulus to adrenaline secretion which directly inhibits breakdown of skeletal muscle.

The liver produces ketone bodies during a very low carb diet and they flow from the liver to extra-hepatic tissues (e.g., brain, muscle) for use as a fuel. In addition, ketone bodies exert a restraining influence on muscle protein breakdown.

During weight loss, higher protein intake reduces loss of muscle mass and increases loss of body fat.

Very-low-carbohydrate diets and preservation of muscle mass. - 2006

Amyotrophic lateral sclerosis (ALS) is an adult-onset neurodegenerative disorder in which spinal and cortical motor neurons die causing relentlessly progressive weakness and wasting of skeletal muscles throughout the body.

Experimental evidence demonstrates that treatment with a ketogenic diet may slow motor deterioration and protect motor neurons through a promoting energy production in the mitochondria of ALS study mice.

A ketogenic diet as a potential novel therapeutic intervention in

30 patients were assigned either an unrestricted diet or instructed to consume less than 20 g of carbohydrates per day for the 1st month and then less than 40 g per day for months 2 and 3.

The dieters lost significantly more weight, but the diet did not increase bone turnover markers compared with controls at any time point.

The effect of a low-carbohydrate diet on bone turnover. - 2006

It is necessary to emphasize that ketogenic diets do not produce osteoporosis.

Ketogenic diets: additional benefits to the weight loss and unfounded secondary effects - 2008

Untrained overweight women were put on either a regular diet or low carb diet, and performed performed 60-100 min of varied resistance exercise twice weekly for 10 weeks.

Subjects on the low carb regime lost ~5.6kg of fat mass with no significant change in lean body mass, while the normal dieters gained ~1.6kg with no significant change in fat mass.

Resistance training in overweight women on a ketogenic diet conserved lean body mass while reducing body fat. - 2010

4 hours following spinal cord injury rats were fed either a standard carbohydrate based diet or a ketogenic diet, and functional recovery was evaluated for 14 weeks.

Ketogenic diet treatment resulted in increased usage and range of motion of the affected forepaw. Furthermore, keto improved pellet retrieval with recovery of wrist and digit movements. Importantly, after returning to a standard diet after 12 weeks of keto treatment, the improved forelimb function remained stable.

The spinal cords of keto treated animals displayed smaller lesion areas and more grey matter sparing.

Post-injury ketogenic diet effectively promotes functional recovery and is neuroprotective after spinal cord injury.

Ketogenic Diet Improves Forelimb Motor Function after Spinal Cord Injury in Rodents. - 2013

The only known treatment of glucose transporter 1 deficiency syndrome is a ketogenic diet, which provides the brain with an alternative fuel, however concerns still remain about its effects on body and bone composition.

In adults with GLUT-1 deficiency syndrome on a ketogenic diet for 5 years there were no appreciable changes in weight and body composition, and no evidence of potential adverse effects on bone health.

Long-term effects of a ketogenic diet on body composition and bone mineralization in GLUT-1 deficiency syndrome: a case series. - 2014

Cancer

Cancer cell growth in culture was inhibited by ketone bodies and this effect was reversible, non-toxic, and proportional to the concentration of ketone bodies. D-beta-hydroxybutyrate was not metabolised by the cells.

Dietary-induced ketosis reduced the number of melanoma deposits in the lungs of mice by two-thirds.

THE INHIBITION OF MALIGNANT CELL GROWTH BY KETONE BODIES. - 1979

An attempt has been made to reverse cachexia (muscle wasting/fatigue/etc) by depriving tumours of energy by feeding a ketogenic regime.

Mice were implanted with a form of colon cancer which produces extensive weight loss without a reduction in food intake.

When mice were fed on diets in which up to 80% of the energy was supplied as medium chain triglycerides (MCT) weight loss was reduced in proportion to the fat content of the diet, and the tumour contributed less to the final body weight.

Reduction of weight loss and tumour size in a cachexia model by a high fat diet. - 1987

2 young girls with brain cancer were put on a ketogenic diet, within a week a decrease of 22% glucose uptake was noted at the sites of the tumor.

One subject continued the ketogenic diet for an additional year, remaining free of disease progression.

Effects of a ketogenic diet on tumor metabolism and nutritional status in pediatric oncology patients: two case reports. - 1995

Normal mammalian brain cells are metabolically versatile and capable of deriving energy from glucose and ketone bodies.

Most tumours including primary brain tumours actively consume glucose and are largely dependent on glycolysis for energy.

Mitochondrial defects and an inability to metabolise ketone bodies are thought to be responsible for the dependence of tumour cells on glycolytic energy.

While this switch occurs readily in normal cells, the switch is more difficult for tumour cells due to their accumulated genetic defects.

We suggest that ketone body metabolism, while providing normal brain cells with an alternative high-energy substrate, also reduces the inflammatory activities of tumour-associated host cells.

A shift in energy metabolism from glucose to ketones will enhance the bioenergetic potential of normal brain cells on the one hand while reducing tumour cell growth and tumour inflammatory properties on the other.

Role of glucose and ketone bodies in the metabolic control of experimental brain cancer. - 2003

As most brain tumour cells are dependent on glycolysis for energy due to mitochondrial defects, they are unable to switch from glucose to ketone bodies for energy.

An energy source shift from glucose to ketone bodies will enhance the bioenergetic potential of normal brain cells while reducing tumour cell growth and tissue inflammation.

Anti-Angiogenic and Pro-Apoptotic Effects of Dietary Restriction in Experimental Brain Cancer: Role of Glucose and Ketone Bodies. - 2005

The role of selected macronutrients, fatty acids and cholesterol in the etiology of prostate cancer was analyzed using data from a case-control study carried out in five Italian areas between 1991 and 2002.

A direct association with prostate cancer was found for starch intake.

Intakes of proteins, sugars, saturated fat, and dietary cholesterol were unrelated to risk.

Macronutrients, fatty acids, cholesterol and prostate cancer risk. - 2005

Adult mice were implanted with malignant brain tumors and put on an either unrestricted or restricted ketogenic diet, the effects on tumor growth, vascularity, and survival were compared with that of an unrestricted high carbohydrate standard diet.

The restricted keto diet reduced glucose levels while elevating ketone body levels, significantly decreased the growth of the tumors, and significantly enhanced health and survival compared to that of the control groups receiving the standard low fat/high carbohydrate diet.

Gene expression was lower in the tumors than in the contralateral normal brain suggesting that these brain tumors have reduced ability to metabolize ketone bodies for energy.

The calorically restricted ketogenic diet, an effective alternative therapy for malignant brain cancer. - 2007

The intake of beef/pork, processed meat, total fat, saturated fat or n-6 PUFA showed no clear association with the overall or subsite-specific risk of colorectal cancer.

These findings do not support the hypothesis that consumption of red meat increases colorectal cancer risk but do suggest that high intake of fish may decrease the risk, particularly of distal colon cancer.

Meat, fish and fat intake in relation to subsite-specific risk of colorectal cancer: The Fukuoka Colorectal Cancer Study. - 2007

Recent evidence suggests carbohydrate intake may influence prostate cancer biology.

In mice injected with cancer, 51 days later mice fed no carbohydrates had tumor volumes 33% smaller than mice on a "Western" diet.

Keto mice had significantly decreased hepatic fatty infiltration.

Dietary treatment was significantly associated with survival, with the longest survival among the ketogenic mice.

Carbohydrate restriction, prostate cancer growth, and the insulin-like growth factor axis. - 2008

Brain tumors are potentially manageable with dietary therapies that lower glucose availability and elevate ketone bodies. These diets target tumor energy metabolism and reduce tumor growth through integrated anti-inflammatory, antiangiogenic, and proapoptotic mechanisms of action.

Targeting energy metabolism in brain cancer with calorically restricted ketogenic diets. - 2008

Seven aggressive human cancer cell lines, and 3 control fibroblast lines were grown in vitro in either glucose, or in glucose plus ketone bodies.

Controls demonstrated normal cell growth, while all cancer lines in ketone bodies demonstrated proportionally inhibited growth.

The results bear on the hypothesized potential for ketogenic diets as therapeutic strategies.

Acetoacetate reduces growth and ATP concentration in cancer cell lines which over-express uncoupling protein 2. - 2009

6 prospective cohort studies with comprehensive dietary assessments, contributing 1,070 cases of colorectal cancer and ~1.5 million person-years of follow-up, were

identified.

The available epidemiologic evidence does not appear to support an independent association between animal fat intake or animal protein intake and colorectal cancer.

Meta-analysis of animal fat or animal protein intake and colorectal cancer.
- 2009

A 65-year-old woman who presented with progressive memory loss, chronic headaches, nausea, and a right hemisphere multi-centric tumor, was put on a calorie restricted ketogenic diet as well as standard therapy.

After two months treatment, the patient's body weight was reduced by about 20% and no discernable brain tumor tissue was detected, biomarker changes showed reduced levels of blood glucose and elevated levels of urinary ketones.

10 weeks after suspension of strict diet therapy MRI evidence of tumor recurrence was found.

Metabolic management of glioblastoma multiforme using standard therapy together with a restricted ketogenic diet: Case Report. - 2010

That there exists an intimate connection between carbohydrates and cancer has been known since the seminal studies performed by different physiologists in the 1920s.

Chronic activation of the IGFR1-IR/PI3K/Akt survival pathway through high blood glucose, insulin and inflammatory cytokines has been proposed as a cause of carcinogenesis and switch towards aerobic glycolysis.

Besides the ability to grow in hypoxic environments, a high glycolytic rate has several additional advantages for the malignant cell.

Increased glucose flux and metabolism promotes several hallmarks of cancer such as excessive proliferation, anti-apoptotic signalling, cell cycle progression and angiogenesis.

With progressive tumorigenesis, cancer cells become more and more 'addicted' to aerobic glycolysis and vulnerable to glucose deprivation. Indeed, several studies have shown that malignant cells in vitro quickly lose ATP and commit apoptosis when starved of glucose

Besides delivering more glucose to the tumor tissue, hyperglycemia has other important negative effects for the host: modest blood glucose elevations as they typically occur after a Western diet meal competitively impair the transport of ascorbic acid into immune cells, so the immune response to malignant cells is diminished.

Hyperglycemia activates inflammatory cytokines that play an important role also for the progression of cancer, high plasma glucose concentrations elevate the levels of circulating insulin and free IGF1, two potent anti-apoptotic and growth factors for most cancer cells

Since 1885, when Ernst Freund described signs of hyperglycemia in 70 out of 70 cancer patients, it has been repeatedly reported that glucose tolerance and insulin sensitivity are diminished in cancer patients even before signs of cachexia (weight loss) become evident

It therefore seems reasonable to assume that dietary carbohydrates mainly fuel malignant cells, while muscle cells are more likely to benefit from an increased fat and protein intake. Most malignant cells lack key mitochondrial enzymes necessary for conversion of ketone bodies and fatty acids to ATP

Evidence has emerged from both animal and laboratory studies indicating that cancer patients could benefit further from a very low carbohydrate ketogenic diet. Under low glucose concentrations, ketone bodies could serve benign cells as a substitute for metabolic demands while offering no such benefit to malign cells.

In 1913 rats with cancer were fed a carbohydrate-free diet, and not only gained more weight than the controls, but also exhibited much less tumor growth and mortality rates, the differences being "... so striking as to leave no room for doubt that the diet was an important factor in enabling the rats to resist the tumor after growth had started."

Another potential benefit of low carbohydrate diets might lie in their influence upon inflammatory processes that take place within various tissues. Inflammation is a well established driver of early tumorigenesis and accompanies most, if not all cancers.

Is There a Role for Carbohydrate Restriction in the Treatment and
Prevention of Cancer? - 2011

As primarily a metabolic disease, malignant brain cancer can be managed through changes in metabolic environment. In contrast to normal neurons and glia, which readily transition to ketone bodies for energy under reduced glucose, malignant brain tumors are strongly dependent on glycolysis for energy.

We propose an alternative approach to brain cancer management that exploits the metabolic flexibility of normal cells at the expense of the genetically defective and metabolically challenged tumor cells. This approach to brain cancer management is supported from recent studies in mice and humans treated with calorie restriction and the ketogenic diet.

Metabolic management of brain cancer. - 2011

Since cancer cells depend on glucose more than normal cells, the effects of low carbohydrate diets to a Western diet on the growth rate of tumors in mice induced with cancer were examined.

To avoid caloric restriction–induced effects, the low carbohydrate diets were isocaloric with the Western diet by increasing protein rather than fat levels because of the reported tumor-promoting effects of high fat and the immune-stimulating effects of high protein.

Tumors appeared in nearly 50% of mice on a Western diet by the age of 1 year whereas no tumors were detected in mice on the low carbohydrate diet.

This difference was associated with weight gains in mice on the Western diet.

Only 1 mouse on the Western diet achieved a normal life span, due to cancer-associated deaths, more than 50% of the mice on the low carbohydrate diet reached or exceeded the normal life span.

A Low Carbohydrate, High Protein Diet Slows Tumor Growth and Prevents Cancer Initiation. - 2011

Following tumor implantation mice were maintained on standard diet or a ketogenic formula.

Keto plus radiation treatment were more than additive, and in 9 of 11 irradiated animals maintained on keto the tumor cells diminished below the level of detection. They were switched to standard diet 101 days after implantation and no signs of tumor recurrence were seen for over 200 days.

The Ketogenic Diet Is an Effective Adjuvant to Radiation Therapy for the Treatment of Malignant Glioma. - 2012

Patients with advanced incurable cancers, normal organ function without diabetes or recent weight loss, and a body mass index of at least 20, were put on a ketogenic diet.

Preliminary data demonstrate that an insulin-inhibiting ketogenic diet is safe and feasible in selected patients with advanced cancer. The extent of ketosis, but not calorie deficit or weight loss, correlated with stable disease or partial remission.

Targeting insulin inhibition as a metabolic therapy in advanced cancer: a pilot safety and feasibility dietary trial in 10 patients. - 2012

Mice transplanted lung cancer were fed a ketogenic diet, combined with radiation resulted in slower tumor growth relative to radiation alone.

These results show that a ketogenic diet enhances radio-chemo-therapy responses in lung cancer xenografts by a mechanism that may involve increased oxidative stress.

Ketogenic Diets Enhance Oxidative Stress and Radio-Chemo-Therapy Responses in Lung Cancer Xenografts. - 2013

In mice with systemic metastatic cancer, a ketogenic diet alone significantly decreased blood glucose, slowed tumor growth, and increased mean survival time by ~57%.

Hyperbaric therapy alone did not influence cancer progression, but combining keto with hyperbaric therapy elicited a significant decrease in blood glucose, tumor growth rate, and a ~78% increase in mean survival time compared to controls.

The Ketogenic Diet and Hyperbaric Oxygen Therapy Prolong Survival in Mice with Systemic Metastatic Cancer. - 2013

Cancer cells express an abnormal metabolism characterized by increased glucose consumption owing to genetic mutations and mitochondrial dysfunction.

Previous studies indicate that unlike healthy tissues, cancer cells are unable to effectively use ketone bodies for energy.

Mice were fed a standard diet supplemented with either 1,3-butanediol or a ketone ester, which are metabolized to ketone bodies.

Ketone supplementation decreased proliferation and viability of the tumor cells grown in vitro, even in the presence of high glucose.

Ketone administration elicited anticancer effects in vitro and in vivo independent of glucose levels or calorie restriction.

Ketone supplementation decreases tumor cell viability and prolongs survival of mice with metastatic cancer - 2014

Aggressive tumors typically demonstrate a high glycolytic rate, which results in resistance to radiation therapy and cancer progression via several molecular and physiologic mechanisms. Intriguingly, many of these mechanisms utilize the same molecular pathways that are altered through calorie and/or carbohydrate restriction.

Important mechanisms include:

- improved DNA repair in normal, but not tumor cells;
- inhibition of tumor cell repopulation;
- redistribution of normal cells into more radioresistant phases of the cell cycle;
- normalization of the tumor vasculature;
- increasing the intrinsic radioresistance of normal cells through ketone bodies but decreasing that of tumor cells by targeting glycolysis.

Calorie restriction and ketogenic diets may act synergistically with radiation therapy for the treatment of cancer patients and provide some guidelines for implementing these dietary interventions into clinical practice.

Calories, carbohydrates, and cancer therapy with radiation: exploiting the five R's through dietary manipulation. - 2014

If cancer is primarily a disease of energy metabolism, then rational strategies for cancer management should be found in those therapies that specifically target tumor cell energy metabolism. As glucose is the major fuel for tumor energy metabolism through lactate fermentation, the restriction of glucose becomes a prime target for management.

It is well known that ketones can replace glucose as an

energy metabolite and can protect the brain from severe hypoglycemia, hence, the shift in energy metabolism associated with a low carbohydrate, high-fat ketogenic diet administered in restricted amounts can protect normal cells from glycolytic inhibition and the brain from hypoglycemia.

When systemic glucose availability becomes limiting, most normal cells of the body will transition their energy metabolism to fats and ketone bodies. Most tumor cells are unable to use ketone bodies for energy due to abnormalities in mitochondria structure or function, ketone bodies can also be toxic to some cancer cells. Nutritional ketosis induces metabolic stress on tumor tissue that is selectively vulnerable to glucose deprivation, hence, metabolic stress will be greater in tumor cells than in normal cells when the whole body is transitioned away from glucose and to ketone bodies for energy.

The metabolic shift from glucose metabolism to ketone body metabolism creates an anti-angiogenic, anti-inflammatory and pro-apoptotic environment within the tumor mass

Cancer as a metabolic disease: implications for novel therapeutics. - 2014

This study assessed the combined association of two factors implicated in breast tumor growth—carbohydrate intake and IGF1 receptor status—to test whether activating the insulin/insulin-like growth-factor axis can impact breast cancer. Since carbohydrates stimulate the biological pathway that can increase concentrations of IGF1, the focus was on carbohydrate intake.

An association was found between increased breast cancer recurrence in women with a primary breast cancer tumor that was positive for the IGF1 receptor and a decreased carbohydrate intake was associated with decreased breast cancer recurrence.

Risk of Breast Cancer Recurrence Associated with Carbohydrate Intake and Tissue Expression of IGF-1 Receptor. - 2014

Organs

To study the metabolic effects of ketosis without weight loss, nine lean men were fed a balanced diet for one week followed by four weeks of a ketogenic diet.

No disturbance of liver or kidney function was noted at the end.

The human metabolic response to chronic ketosis without caloric restriction: physical and biochemical adaptation. - 1983

51 obese people with healthy gallbladders were put on a severely restricted practically fat-free diet of 500 calories a day.

After 4 weeks, 4 subjects had developed gall stones and 1 subject revealed gallbladder sludge.

After 8 weeks and ~16kg of bodyweight loss, 13 of them had developed gall stones and one subject required removal of the gallbladder, with two further cases requiring removal some time after the intervention period.

6 months later 4 of the subjects gallstones had disappeared.

Gallstone formation during weight-reduction dieting. - 1989

Gallstone-free obese subjects were placed on severely restricted diets with either 3g or 12g of fat per day.

Over half of the subjects in the lower fat group who

completed the study developed gallstones, whereas none of the subjects in the "higher" fat group suffered such a fate.

Gallbladder motility and gallstone formation in obese patients following very low calorie diets. Use it (fat) to lose it (well). - 1998

65 healthy overweight/obese subjects were put on ad libitum low fat diets with protein intake either low or moderate for 6 months.

Kidney volume and glomerular filtration rate decreased on the low protein diet, and increased in the moderate protein group. Albuminuria remained unchanged in both groups.

Moderate changes in dietary protein intake cause adaptive alterations in renal size and function to suit needs, without indications of adverse effects.

Changes in renal function during weight loss induced by high vs low-protein low-fat diets in overweight subjects. - 1999

In a rats heart ketones increased contractility and decreased oxygen consumption, and decreased the death of lung cells induced by hemorrhagic shock.

Ketoacids? Good medicine? - 2003

A high intake of carbohydrates increases the risk of symptomatic gall stone disease in men. These results add to the concern that low fat high carbohydrate diets may not be an optimal dietary recommendation.

Dietary carbohydrates and glycaemic load and the incidence of
symptomatic gall stone disease in men. - 2005

While protein restriction may be appropriate for treatment of existing kidney disease, there is no significant evidence for a detrimental effect of high protein intakes on kidney function in healthy persons after centuries of a high protein Western diet.

Dietary protein intake and renal function. - 2005

91 patients with non-alcoholic fatty liver disease - 31 with metabolic syndrome - completed a food frequency questionnaire.

Patients with metabolic syndrome had a higher HOMA index, scores for steatosis, NASH activity, global NASH score, and and consumed more carbohydrates and less fat.

Metabolic syndrome is associated with greater histologic severity, higher
carbohydrate, and lower fat diet in patients with NAFLD. - 2006

An obese patient with type 2 diabetes whose diet was changed from the recommended high-carbohydrate, low-fat type to a low-carbohydrate diet demonstrated reversal of a 6 year long decline of renal function.

A low-carbohydrate diet may prevent end-stage renal failure in type 2
diabetes. A case report. - 2006

5 patients with a mean BMI of ~36 and fatty liver disease were instructed to follow a ketogenic diet with nutritional supplementation for 6 months.

4 of 5 post-treatment liver biopsies showed histologic improvements in steatosis, inflammatory grade, and fibrosis.

The Effect of a Low-Carbohydrate, Ketogenic Diet on Nonalcoholic Fatty Liver Disease: A Pilot Study. - 2007

64 obese diabetic subjects were put on a ketogenic diet and monitored for 56 weeks, the changes in the level of by-products indicating renal function were not statistically significant.

Beneficial effects of ketogenic diet in obese diabetic subjects. - 2007

Renal function was assessed in 68 men and women with abdominal obesity without preexisting renal dysfunction who were randomized to consume either an energy-restricted very-low-carbohydrate or high-carbohydrate diet for 1 year.

There were no changes in either group in serum creatinine levels or estimated glomerular filtration rate.

Renal function following long-term weight loss in individuals with abdominal obesity on a very-low-carbohydrate diet vs high-carbohydrate diet. - 2010

Intensive insulin therapy and protein restriction delay the development of nephropathy (kidney disease) in a variety of conditions, but few interventions are known to reverse nephropathy.

In mouse models diabetic nephropathy was allowed to develop, then half the mice were switched to a ketogenic diet. After 8 weeks it was completely reversed.

Reversal of Diabetic Nephropathy by a Ketogenic Diet. - 2011

A prospective study was carried out in 14 obese men with nonalcoholic fatty liver disease, advised to undertake a Spanish Ketogenic Mediterranean Diet.

Complete fatty liver regression was observed in ~21% of the patients, and an overall reduction was found in ~93%.

The effect of the Spanish Ketogenic Mediterranean Diet on nonalcoholic fatty liver disease: a pilot study - 2011

307 obese adults without serious medical illnesses were randomly assigned to a low-carbohydrate high-protein or a low-fat weight-loss diet for 24 months.

There was no noticeably harmful effects on kidney function compared with a low-fat diet.

Comparative effects of low-carbohydrate high-protein versus low-fat diets on the kidney. - 2012

Hormones

The effect of varying carbohydrate intake upon plasma insulin and glucagon was tested in five volunteers.

One week of carbohydrate restriction lowered fasting insulin, whereas fasting glucagon rose, with a decline in insulin-glucagon ratio (I/G), and changed the response of insulin and glucagon to protein, insulin rising only small amounts, whereas glucagon rose significantly.

One week of restoration of carbohydrate to the diet increased fasting insulin and reduced glucagon, the I/G ratio returning to "normal", insulin rising significantly and glucagon only a little, with I/G ratio rising significantly.

The Influence of the Antecedent Diet upon Glucagon and Insulin Secretion.
- 1971

A test meal containing gelatin plus glucose resulted in much higher levels of insulin and I/G, lower glucagon levels than a meal of the same size of gelatin alone.

One week of a 12 g/day carbohydrate, 2870 calorie diet lowered insulin, I/G, plus increased glucagon.

A 390 g/day carbohydrate, 2784-calorie intake significantly increased insulin, I/G, and lowered glucagon within two days; even greater changes in hormones were observed on a 510 g/day carbohydrate intake.

Basal and postprotein insulin and glucagon levels during a high and low carbohydrate intake and their relationships to plasma triglycerides. - 1975

During a ketogenic regimen concentrations of fat derived substrates rise significantly and glucose levels decrease, hormonal patterns switch towards a catabolic mode with a fall in insulin levels and a rise in glucagon concentration, levels of gluconeogenic amino acids are reduced while those of the branched chain amino acids increase.

These changes also reproduce those observed after a few days of total fasting, suggesting it is the carbohydrate restriction itself which is responsible.

Hormonal and metabolic changes induced by an isocaloric isoproteinic ketogenic diet in healthy subjects. - 1982

8 healthy untrained men aged ~22 spent 3 days on a ketogenic diet, both the pre-and post-exercise levels of adrenaline, noradrenaline, and cortisol were enhanced, whilst plasma insulin concentration was decreased.

Effect of low-carbohydrate-ketogenic diet on metabolic and hormonal responses to graded exercise in men. - 1996

After intake of high-carbohydrate meal, overweight men had higher hyperinsulinemia than did the lean men.

Postprandial de novo lipogenesis and metabolic changes induced by a high-carbohydrate, low-fat meal in lean and overweight men. - 2001

Testosterone, cortisol, and insulin responses to a high-fat test meal were determined before and after an 8-week high-fat diet in 11 healthy men.

The high-fat diet resulted in significant reductions in insulin, with no significant changes in testosterone and cortisol. However for 8 hours following a high fat meal testosterone and cortisol levels were reduced.

Effects of a high-fat diet on postabsorptive and postprandial testosterone responses to a fat-rich meal. - 2001

There were significant decreases in fasting serum insulin concentrations after men consumed the ketogenic diet.

A Ketogenic Diet Favorably Affects Serum Biomarkers for Cardiovascular Disease in Normal-Weight Men. - 2002

12 healthy normal-weight men switched from their habitual diet to a carbohydrate-restricted diet for 6 weeks, there was a significant decrease in serum insulin, and an increase in total thyroxine (thyroid hormone).

Body composition and hormonal responses to a carbohydrate-restricted diet. - 2002

11 obese women were randomly assigned to a 10 week dietary intervention study comparing high protein or high carb energy restricted diets, a significant decrease in fasting leptin in the high protein group.

Effects of protein vs. carbohydrate-rich diets on fuel utilisation in obese women during weight loss. - 2003

Severely obese subjects were assigned to a carbohydrate-restricted or a calorie- and fat-restricted diet.

Insulin sensitivity improved more among subjects on the low-carbohydrate diet.

A Low-Carbohydrate as Compared with a Low-Fat Diet in Severe Obesity. - 2003

53 obese females were randomized to either a low-fat restricted calorie diet, or a low-carbohydrate unrestricted calorie diet.

The women in the very low carbohydrate group maintained normal levels of insulin.

A Randomized Trial Comparing a Very Low Carbohydrate Diet and a Calorie-Restricted Low Fat Diet on Body Weight and Cardiovascular Risk Factors in Healthy Women. - 2003

11 women with a BMI >27 and a clinical diagnosis of PCOS were instructed to limit their carbohydrate intake to 20 grams or less per day for 24 weeks.

There were statistically significant reductions in percent free testosterone, LH/FSH ratio, and fasting serum insulin.

The effects of a low-carbohydrate, ketogenic diet on the polycystic ovary syndrome: a pilot study. - 2005

55 people of ~33 BMI were put on diets restricted by

~500 calories for 4 months, of either 1.6g/kg protein and <170g carbohydrate, or 0.8g/kg protein and >220g carbohydrate.

Insulin responses to the meal challenge were significantly improved in lower compared to higher carb at both 1 and 2 hours.

Moderate carbohydrate, moderate protein weight loss diet reduces cardiovascular disease risk compared to high carbohydrate, low protein diet in obese adults: A randomized clinical trial. - 2008

Subjects with atherogenic dyslipidemia were examined on a 12-week study of a ~1,500 kcal carbohydrate-restricted diet, experiencing significantly reduced insulin, and insulin sensitivity improvements.

Carbohydrate Restriction has a More Favorable Impact on the Metabolic Syndrome than a Low Fat Diet. - 2009

Ketogenic mice experienced substantially reduced insulin even in the absence of weight loss.

A very low carbohydrate ketogenic diet improves glucose tolerance in ob/ob mice independently of weight loss. - 2009

The circulating concentrations of several hormones and nutrients which influence appetite were altered after weight loss induced by a ketogenic diet, compared with after refeeding.

When participants were ketotic, the weight loss induced

increase in ghrelin was suppressed. Amylin and leptin were lower at week 8 than after refeeding.

Ketosis and appetite-mediating nutrients and hormones after weight loss. - 2013

Carbohydrates Role In Human Nutrition

There is no clear requirement for dietary carbohydrates for human adults.

Current carbohydrate recommendations are based on:

1. preventing ketosis
2. providing glucose beyond minimal needs

However, it is clear that ketosis is not harmful.

The need to provide glucose above minimal needs is exactly what has never been demonstrated.

The National Research Council has not established Recommended Dietary Allowance (RDA) for carbohydrates, probably because the human body can adapt to a carbohydrate-free diet and manufacture the glucose it needs.

Metabolic Effects of the Very-Low-Carbohydrate Diets: Misunderstood "Villains" of Human Metabolism. - 2004

Glucose is essential only in a few organs: the brain, the kidney (medulla) and the red blood cells.

In the absence of dietary carbohydrate, the body is able to synthesize glucose from lactic acid, certain amino acids and glycerol via gluconeogenesis.

Essentials of Human Nutrition - 2007

The lower limit of dietary carbohydrate compatible with life apparently is zero, provided that adequate amounts of protein and fat are consumed.

Dietary Guidelines for Americans - 2010

Carbohydrates are not essential nutrients.

Lecture Notes: Clinical Biochemistry - 2011

No specific carbohydrates have been identified as dietary requirements.

Marks' Basic Medical Biochemistry - 2012

Carbohydrates are not essential nutrients.

Biochemistry - 2013

References

The use of a high fat diet in the treatment of diabetes mellitus: First paper - 1920
NEWBURGH LH & MARSH PL, 1920.
Archives of Internal Medicine, 26(6), pp.647–662.
Available at: http://dx.doi.org/10.1001/archinte.1920.00100060002001

The use of a high fat diet in the treatment of diabetes mellitus: Second paper: blood sugar. - 1921
NEWBURGH LH & MARSH PL, 1921.
Archives of Internal Medicine, 27(6), pp.699–705.
Available at: http://dx.doi.org/10.1001/archinte.1921.00100120070005

An Experience with a Ketogenic Dietary in Migraine
SCHNABEL, T.G., 1928.
Annals of Internal Medicine, 2(4), pp.341–347.
Available at: http://dx.doi.org/10.7326/0003-4819-2-4-341

The Effect of an Exclusive Meat Diet on the Chemical Constituents of the Blood. - 1929
Tolstoi, E., 1929.
Journal of Biological Chemistry, 83(3), pp.753–758.
Available at: http://www.jbc.org/content/83/3/753

The Treatment of Obesity: A Comparison of the Effects of Diet and of Thyroid Extract. - 1932
Lyon, D.M. & Dunlop, D.M., 1932.
QJM, 1(2), pp.331–352.
Available at: http://qjmed.oxfordjournals.org/content/1/2/331

THE GLYCEMIC RESPONSE TO ISOGLUCOGENIC QUANTITIES OF PROTEIN AND CARBOHYDRATE. - 1936
Conn, J.W. & Newburgh, L.H., 1936.
Journal of Clinical Investigation, 15(6), pp.665–671.
Available at: http://www.jci.org/articles/view/100818

RESULTS OF 15 YEARS' EXPERIENCE WITH THE KETOGENIC DIET IN THE TREATMENT OF EPILEPSY IN CHILDREN. - 1938
Helmholz, H.F. & Goldstein, M., 1938.
American Journal of Psychiatry, 94(5), pp.1205–1214.
Available at: http://ajp.psychiatryonline.org/article.aspx?articleID=141440

Diet and the Genesis of Diabetes Mellitus - 1947

Anon, 1947.
Acta Medica Scandinavica, 128(S198), pp.1–14.
Available at: http://onlinelibrary.wiley.com/doi/10.1111/j.0954-6820.1947.tb13795.x/abstract

Treatment of OBESITY with Calorically UNRESTRICTED DIETS. - 1953
Pennington, A.W., 1953.
The American Journal of Clinical Nutrition, 1(5), pp.343–348.
Available at: http://ajcn.nutrition.org/content/1/5/343

Calorie intake in relation to body-weight changes in the obese. - 1956
Kekwick, A. & Pawan, G.L., 1956.
Lancet, 271(6935), pp.155–161.
Available at: http://www.ncbi.nlm.nih.gov/pubmed/13347103

Ketosis, weight loss, uric acid, and nitrogen balance in obese women fed single nutrients at low caloric levels - 1969
Bell, J.D., Margen, S. & Calloway, D.H., 1969.
Metabolism - Clinical and Experimental, 18(3), pp.193–208.
Available at:
http://www.metabolismjournal.com/article/0026049569900390/abstract

Nutrient Intake of Subjects on Low Carbohydrate Diet Used in Treatment of Obesity. - 1970
Stock, A.L. & Yudkin, J., 1970.
The American Journal of Clinical Nutrition, 23(7), pp.948–952.
Available at: http://ajcn.nutrition.org/content/23/7/948

The Influence of the Antecedent Diet upon Glucagon and Insulin Secretion. - 1971
Muller, W.A., Faloona, G.R. & Unger, R.H., 1971.
New England Journal of Medicine, 285(26), pp.1450–1454.
Available at: http://www.nejm.org/doi/full/10.1056/NEJM197112232852603

Effect on body composition and other parameters in obese young men of carbohydrate level of reduction diet. - 1971
Young, C.M. et al., 1971.
The American Journal of Clinical Nutrition, 24(3), pp.290–296.
Available at: http://ajcn.nutrition.org/content/24/3/290

Resistance to symptomatic insulin reactions after fasting. - 1972
Drenick, E.J. et al., 1972.
The Journal of clinical investigation, 51(10), pp.2757–2762.
Available at: http://www.ncbi.nlm.nih.gov/pubmed/5056667/

Response of body weight to a low carbohydrate, high fat diet in normal and obese subjects. - 1973
Kasper, H., Thiel, H. & Ehl, M., 1973.
The American Journal of Clinical Nutrition, 26(2), pp.197–204.
Available at: http://ajcn.nutrition.org/content/26/2/197

The Absence of Undesirable Changes during Consumption of the Low Carbohydrate Diet. - 1974
Evans, E., Stock, A.L. & Yudkin, J., 1974.
Annals of Nutrition and Metabolism, 17(6), pp.360–367.
Available at: https://www.karger.com/Article/Abstract/175560

Exercise-induced increase in the capacity of rat skeletal muscle to oxidize ketones. - 1975
Winder, W.W., Baldwin, K.M. & Holloszy, J.O., 1975.
Canadian journal of physiology and pharmacology, 53(1), pp.86–91.
Available at: http://www.ncbi.nlm.nih.gov/pubmed/237626

Basal and postprotein insulin and glucagon levels during a high and low carbohydrate intake and their relationships to plasma triglycerides. - 1975
Fukita, Y., Gott o, A.M. & Unger, R.H., 1975.
Diabetes, 24(6), pp.552–558.
Available at: http://www.ncbi.nlm.nih.gov/pubmed/1095439

Isocaloric diet changes and electroencephalographic sleep. - 1975
Phillips, F. et al., 1975.
Lancet, 2(7938), pp.723–725.
Available at: http://www.ncbi.nlm.nih.gov/pubmed/52766

Effect of diet composition on metabolic adaptations to hypocaloric nutrition: comparison of high carbohydrate and high fat isocaloric diets. - 1977
Lewis, S.B. et al., 1977.
The American Journal of Clinical Nutrition, 30(2), pp.160–170.
Available at: http://www.ncbi.nlm.nih.gov/pubmed/835502

Hematological and metabolic responses to training in racing sled dogs fed diets containing medium, low, or zero carbohydrate. - 1977
Kronfeld, D.S. et al., 1977.
The American Journal of Clinical Nutrition, 30(3), pp.419–430.
Available at: http://www.ncbi.nlm.nih.gov/pubmed/842493

Chronic ketosis and cerebral metabolism. - 1978
DeVivo, D.C. et al., 1978.

Annals of neurology, 3(4), pp.331–337.
Available at: http://www.ncbi.nlm.nih.gov/pubmed/666275

Effect of a high protein (meat) intake on calcium metabolism in man. - 1978
Spencer, H. et al., 1978.
The American Journal of Clinical Nutrition, 31(12), pp.2167–2180.
Available at: http://www.ncbi.nlm.nih.gov/pubmed/727162

Comparative studies in obese subjects fed carbohydrate-restricted and high carbohydrate 1,000-calorie formula diets. - 1978
Rabast, U., Kasper, H. & Schönborn, J., 1978.
Nutrition and Metabolism, 22(5), pp.269–277.
Available at: http://www.ncbi.nlm.nih.gov/pubmed/662209

Dietetic treatment of obesity with low and high-carbohydrate diets: comparative studies and clinical results. - 1979
Rabast, U., Schönborn, J. & Kasper, H., 1979.
International journal of obesity, 3(3), pp.201–211.
Available at: http://www.ncbi.nlm.nih.gov/pubmed/395115

THE INHIBITION OF MALIGNANT CELL GROWTH BY KETONE BODIES. - 1979
Magee et al, 1979.
Immunology and Cell Biology, Aust J Exp Biol Med, 57(5), pp.529–539.
Available   at:
http://www.nature.com/icb/journal/v57/n5/abs/icb197954a.html

Effects of high-protein, low-carbohydrate dieting on plasma lipoproteins and body weight. - 1980
Larosa, J.C. et al., 1980.
Journal of the American Dietetic Association, 77(3), pp.264–270.
Available at: http://www.ncbi.nlm.nih.gov/pubmed/7410754

Capacity for Moderate Exercise in Obese Subjects after Adaptation to a Hypocaloric, Ketogenic Diet. - 1980
Phinney, S.D. et al., 1980.
Journal of Clinical Investigation, 66(5), pp.1152–1161.
Available at: http://www.jci.org/articles/view/109945

Loss of weight, sodium and water in obese persons consuming a high- or low-carbohydrate diet. - 1981
Rabast, U., Vornberger, K.H. & Ehl, M., 1981.
Annals of nutrition & metabolism, 25(6), pp.341–349.
Available at: http://www.ncbi.nlm.nih.gov/pubmed/7332312

Respiratory failure precipitated by high carbohydrate loads. - 1981
Covelli, H.D. et al., 1981.
Annals of Internal Medicine, 95(5), pp.579–581.
Available at: http://www.ncbi.nlm.nih.gov/pubmed/6794409

The regulation of ketogenesis. - 1982
Foster, D.W. & McGarry, J.D., 1982.
Ciba Foundation symposium, 87, pp.120–131.
Available at: http://www.ncbi.nlm.nih.gov/pubmed/6122545

Hormonal and metabolic changes induced by an isocaloric isoproteinic ketogenic diet in healthy subjects. - 1982
Fery, F. et al., 1982.
Diabète & métabolisme, 8(4), pp.299–305.
Available at: http://www.ncbi.nlm.nih.gov/pubmed/6761185

Post-exercise ketosis and the hormone response to exercise: a review. - 1982
Koeslag, J.H., 1982.
Medicine and science in sports and exercise, 14(5), pp.327–334.
Availble at: http://www.ncbi.nlm.nih.gov/pubmed/6759842

Further studies of the effect of a high protein diet as meat on calcium metabolism. 1983
Spencer, H. et al., 1983.
The American Journal of Clinical Nutrition, 37(6), pp.924–929.
Available at: http://ajcn.nutrition.org/content/37/6/924.abstract

The human metabolic response to chronic ketosis without caloric restriction: preservation of submaximal exercise capability with reduced carbohydrate oxidation. - 1983
Phinney, S.D. et al., 1983.
Metabolism: Clinical and Experimental, 32(8), pp.769–776.
Available at: http://www.ncbi.nlm.nih.gov/pubmed/6865776

The human metabolic response to chronic ketosis without caloric restriction: physical and biochemical adaptation. - 1983
Phinney, S.D. et al., 1983.
Metabolism: clinical and experimental, 32(8), pp.757–768.
Available at: http://www.ncbi.nlm.nih.gov/pubmed/6865775

Adaptation to overeating in lean and overweight men and women. - 1983
Webb, P. & Annis, J.F., 1983.
Human Nutrition. Clinical Nutrition, 37(2), pp.117–131.
Available at: http://www.ncbi.nlm.nih.gov/pubmed/6575005

The effects of high-carbohydrate and high-fat diets on the serum lipid and lipoprotein concentrations of endurance athletes. - 1984

Thompson, P.D. et al., 1984.
Metabolism: Clinical and Experimental, 33(11), pp.1003–1010.
Available at: http://www.ncbi.nlm.nih.gov/pubmed/6436637

A commentary on the Rationale of the Diet-Heart Statement of the American Heart Association. - 1984

Reiser, R., 1984.
The American Journal of Clinical Nutrition, 40(3), pp.654–658.
Available at: http://www.ncbi.nlm.nih.gov/pubmed/6383010

Hypoxia induced preferential ketone utilization by rat brain slices. - 1984

Kirsch, J.R. & D'Alecy, L.G., 1984.
Stroke; a journal of cerebral circulation, 15(2), pp.319–323.
Available at: http://www.ncbi.nlm.nih.gov/pubmed/6422588

Adaptations to a high-fat diet that increase exercise endurance in male rats. - 1984

Miller, W.C., Bryce, G.R. & Conlee, R.K., 1984.
Journal of Applied Physiology: Respiratory, Environmental and Exercise Physiology, 56(1), pp.78–83.
Available at: http://www.ncbi.nlm.nih.gov/pubmed/6693336

Effects of a low carbohydrate isoenergetic diet on sleep behavior and pulmonary functions in healthy female adult humans. - 1986

Kwan, R.M., Thomas, S. & Mir, M.A., 1986.
The Journal of Nutrition, 116(12), pp.2393–2402.
Available at: http://www.ncbi.nlm.nih.gov/pubmed/3100737

Deleterious metabolic effects of high-carbohydrate, sucrose-containing diets in patients with non-insulin-dependent diabetes mellitus. - 1987

Coulston, A.M. et al., 1987.
The American Journal of Medicine, 82(2), pp.213–220.
Available at: http://www.ncbi.nlm.nih.gov/pubmed/3544839

Reduction of weight loss and tumour size in a cachexia model by a high fat diet. - 1987

Tisdale, M.J., Brennan, R.A. & Fearon, K.C., 1987.
British journal of cancer, 56(1), pp.39–43.
Available at: http://www.ncbi.nlm.nih.gov/pubmed/3620317

Reducing the serum cholesterol level with a diet high in animal fat. - 1988

Newbold, H.L., 1988.
Southern Medical Journal, 81(1), pp.61–63.
Available at: http://www.ncbi.nlm.nih.gov/pubmed/3336803

Comparison of a High-Carbohydrate Diet with a High-Monounsaturated-Fat Diet in Patients with Non-Insulin-Dependent Diabetes Mellitus. - 1988
Garg, A. et al., 1988.
New England Journal of Medicine, 319(13), pp.829–834.
Available at: http://www.nejm.org/doi/pdf/10.1056/NEJM198809293191304

Persistence of Hypertriglyceridemic Effect of Low-Fat High-Carbohydrate Diets in NIDDM Patients. - 1989
Coulston, A.M. et al., 1989.
Diabetes Care, 12(2), pp.94–101.
Available at: http://care.diabetesjournals.org/content/12/2/94

Gallstone formation during weight-reduction dieting. - 1989
Liddle, R.A., Goldstein, R.B. & Saxton, J., 1989.
Archives of Internal Medicine, 149(8), pp.1750–1753.
Available at: http://www.ncbi.nlm.nih.gov/pubmed/2669662

Influence of dietary carbohydrate-to-fat ratio on whole body nitrogen retention and body composition in adult rats. - 1989
McCargar, L.J., Baracos, V.E. & Clandinin, M.T., 1989.
The Journal of nutrition, 119(9), pp.1240–1245.
Available at: http://www.ncbi.nlm.nih.gov/pubmed/2795238

Glycogen repletion and exercise endurance in rats adapted to a high fat diet - 1990
Conlee, R.K. et al., 1990.
Metabolism: clinical and experimental, 39(3), pp.289–294.
Available at: http://www.ncbi.nlm.nih.gov/pubmed/2300519/

Additive effects of training and high-fat diet on energy metabolism during exercise - 1991
Simi, B. et al., 1991.
Journal of applied physiology (Bethesda, Md.: 1985), 71(1), pp.197–203.
Available at: http://www.ncbi.nlm.nih.gov/pubmed/1917743/

Effect of 3-hydroxybutyrate on posttraumatic metabolism in man. - 1991
A, H. et al., 1991.
Surgery, 109(2), pp.176–181.
Available at: http://europepmc.org/abstract/MED/1992551

The transient hypercholesterolemia of major weight loss. - 1991
Phinney, S.D. et al., 1991.
The American journal of clinical nutrition, 53(6), pp.1404–1410.
Available at: http://www.ncbi.nlm.nih.gov/pubmed/2035468

Ketone infusion lowers hormonal responses to hypoglycaemia: evidence for acute cerebral utilization of a non-glucose fuel - 1991
Amiel, S.A. et al., 1991.
Clinical science (London, England: 1979), 81(2), pp.189–194.
Available at: http://www.ncbi.nlm.nih.gov/pubmed/1653662

A high-monounsaturated-fat/low-carbohydrate diet improves peripheral insulin sensitivity in non-insulin-dependent diabetic patients. - 1992
Parillo, M. et al., 1992.
Metabolism, 41(12), pp.1373–1378.
Available at: http://www.ncbi.nlm.nih.gov/pubmed/1461145

Comparison of Effects of High and Low Carbohydrate Diets on Plasma Lipoproteins and Insulin Sensitivity in Patients With Mild NIDDM. - 1992
Garg, A., Grundy, S.M. & Unger, R.H., 1992.
Diabetes, 41(10), pp.1278–1285.
Available at: http://www.ncbi.nlm.nih.gov/pubmed/1397701

Carbohydrate restriction regulates the adaptive response to fasting. - 1992
Klein, S. & Wolfe, R.R., 1992.
The American Journal of Physiology, 262(5 Pt 1), pp.E631–636.
Available at: http://www.ncbi.nlm.nih.gov/pubmed/1590373

Effect of dietary fat on metabolic adjustments to maximal VO2 and endurance in runners. - 1994
Muoio, D.M. et al., 1994.
Medicine and Science in Sports and Exercise, 26(1), pp.81–88.
Available at: http://www.ncbi.nlm.nih.gov/pubmed/8133743

Enhanced endurance in trained cyclists during moderate intensity exercise following 2 weeks adaptation to a high fat diet. - 1994
Lambert, E.V. et al., 1994.
European journal of applied physiology and occupational physiology, 69(4), pp.287–293.
Available at: http://www.ncbi.nlm.nih.gov/pubmed/7851362

Effects of varying carbohydrate content of diet in patients with non—insulin-dependent diabetes mellitus. - 1994

Garg A et al., 1994.
JAMA, 271(18), pp.1421–1428.
Available at: http://www.ncbi.nlm.nih.gov/pubmed/7848401

Hypocaloric high-protein diet improves glucose oxidation and spares lean body mass: comparison to hypocaloric high-carbohydrate diet. - 1994
Piatti, P.M. et al., 1994.
Metabolism: Clinical and Experimental, 43(12), pp.1481–1487.
Available at: http://www.ncbi.nlm.nih.gov/pubmed/7990700

Effects of a ketogenic diet on tumor metabolism and nutritional status in pediatric oncology patients: two case reports. - 1995
Nebeling, L.C. et al., 1995.
Journal of the American College of Nutrition, 14(2), pp.202–208.
Available at: http://www.ncbi.nlm.nih.gov/pubmed/7790697

Potential role of raising dietary protein intake for reducing risk of atherosclerosis. - 1995
Wolfe, B.M., 1995.
The Canadian Journal of Cardiology, 11 Suppl G, p.127G–131G.
Available at: http://www.ncbi.nlm.nih.gov/pubmed/7585287

Effects of unbalanced diets on cerebral glucose metabolism in the adult rat. - 1995
al-Mudallal, A.S. et al., 1995.
Neurology, 45(12), pp.2261–2265.
Available at: http://www.ncbi.nlm.nih.gov/pubmed/8848204

Effect of low-carbohydrate-ketogenic diet on metabolic and hormonal responses to graded exercise in men. - 1996
Langfort, J. et al., 1996.
Journal of Physiology and Pharmacology: An Official Journal of the Polish Physiological Society, 47(2), pp.361–371.
Available at: http://www.ncbi.nlm.nih.gov/pubmed/8807563

Comparison of nutrient intake among depressed and nondepressed individuals. - 1996
Christensen, L. & Somers, S., 1996.
The International Journal of Eating Disorders, 20(1), pp.105–109.
Available at: http://www.ncbi.nlm.nih.gov/pubmed/8807358

Early insulin and glucagon responses to different food items. - 1996
LeBlanc, J., Soucy, J. & Nadeau, A., 1996.
Hormone and metabolic research = Hormon- und Stoffwechselforschung = Hormones et métabolisme, 28(6), pp.276–279.

Available at: http://www.ncbi.nlm.nih.gov/pubmed/8811328

The low fat/low cholesterol diet is ineffective. - 1997
Corr, L.A. & Oliver, M.F., 1997.
European heart journal, 18(1), pp.18–22.
Available at: http://www.ncbi.nlm.nih.gov/pubmed/9049510

The effects of a high-protein, low-fat, ketogenic diet on adolescents with morbid obesity: body composition, blood chemistries, and sleep abnormalities. - 1998
Willi, S.M. et al., 1998.
Pediatrics, 101(1 Pt 1), pp.61–67.
Available at: http://www.ncbi.nlm.nih.gov/pubmed/9417152

The questionable role of saturated and polyunsaturated fatty acids in cardiovascular disease. - 1998
Ravnskov, U., 1998.
Journal of Clinical Epidemiology, 51(6), pp.443–460.
Available at: http://www.ncbi.nlm.nih.gov/pubmed/9635993

Gallbladder motility and gallstone formation in obese patients following very low calorie diets. Use it (fat) to lose it (well). - 1998
Festi, D. et al., 1998.
International Journal of Obesity and Related Metabolic Disorders: Journal of the International Association for the Study of Obesity, 22(6), pp.592–600.
Available at: www.ncbi.nlm.nih.gov/pubmed/9665682

Alterations in mood after changing to a low-fat diet. - 1998
Wells, A.S. et al., 1998.
The British Journal of Nutrition, 79(1), pp.23–30.
Available at: http://www.ncbi.nlm.nih.gov/pubmed/9505799

The efficacy of the ketogenic diet-1998: a prospective evaluation of intervention in 150 children. - 1998
Freeman, J.M. et al., 1998.
Pediatrics, 102(6), pp.1358–1363.
Available at: http://www.ncbi.nlm.nih.gov/pubmed/9832569

The effects of carbohydrate restriction in patients with diet-controlled gestational diabetes. - 1998
Major, C.A. et al., 1998.
Obstetrics and Gynecology, 91(4), pp.600–604.
Available at: http://www.ncbi.nlm.nih.gov/pubmed/9540949

A multicenter study of the efficacy of the ketogenic diet. - 1998
Vining, E.P. et al., 1998.
Archives of neurology, 55(11), pp.1433–1437.
Available at: http://www.ncbi.nlm.nih.gov/pubmed/9823827/

Utility of a short-term 25% carbohydrate diet on improving glycemic control in type 2 diabetes mellitus. - 1998
Gutierrez, M. et al., 1998.
Journal of the American College of Nutrition, 17(6), pp.595–600.
Available at: http://www.ncbi.nlm.nih.gov/pubmed/9853539

Metabolic adaptations to a high-fat diet in endurance cyclists - 1999
Goedecke, J.H. et al., 1999.
Metabolism: clinical and experimental, 48(12), pp.1509–1517.
Available at: http://www.ncbi.nlm.nih.gov/pubmed/10599981

Changes in renal function during weight loss induced by high vs low-protein low-fat diets in overweight subjects. - 1999
Skov, A.R. et al., 1999.
International Journal of Obesity and Related Metabolic Disorders: Journal of the International Association for the Study of Obesity, 23(11), pp.1170–1177.
Available at: http://www.ncbi.nlm.nih.gov/pubmed/10578207

Randomized trial on protein vs carbohydrate in ad libitum fat reduced diet for the treatment of obesity. - 1999
Skov, A.R. et al., 1999.
International Journal of Obesity and Related Metabolic Disorders: Journal of the International Association for the Study of Obesity, 23(5), pp.528–536.
Available at: http://www.ncbi.nlm.nih.gov/pubmed/10375057

Fasting lipoprotein and postprandial triglyceride responses to a low-carbohydrate diet supplemented with n-3 fatty acids. - 2000
Volek, J.S., Gómez, A.L. & Kraemer, W.J., 2000.
Journal of the American College of Nutrition, 19(3), pp.383–391.
Available at: http://www.ncbi.nlm.nih.gov/pubmed/10872901

Treatment of hypertriglyceridemia by two diets rich either in unsaturated fatty acids or in carbohydrates: effects on lipoprotein subclasses, lipolytic enzymes, lipid transfer proteins, insulin and leptin. - 2000
Pieke, B. et al., 2000.
International Journal of Obesity and Related Metabolic Disorders: Journal of the International Association for the Study of Obesity, 24(10), pp.1286–1296.
Available at: http://www.ncbi.nlm.nih.gov/pubmed/11093290

Metabolic and Anthropometric changes in obese subjects from an unrestricted calorie, high monounsaturated fat, very low carbohydrate diet. - 2000
Goldberg, J.M. & O'Mara, K., 2000.
Journal of Clinical Ligand Assay, 23(2), pp.97–103.
Available at: http://www.cabdirect.org/abstracts/20013131121.html

d-β-Hydroxybutyrate protects neurons in models of Alzheimer's and Parkinson's disease - 2000
Kashiwaya, Y. et al., 2000.
Proceedings of the National Academy of Sciences, 97(10), pp.5440–5444.
Available at: http://www.pnas.org/content/97/10/5440

The impact of egg limitations on coronary heart disease risk: do the numbers add up? - 2000
McNamara, D.J., 2000.
Journal of the American College of Nutrition, 19(5 Suppl), p.540S–548S.
Available at: http://www.ncbi.nlm.nih.gov/pubmed/11023005

Fat utilization during exercise: adaptation to a fat-rich diet increases utilization of plasma fatty acids and very low density lipoprotein-triglyceride in humans. - 2001
Helge, J.W. et al., 2001.
The Journal of Physiology, 537(3), pp.1009–1020.
Available at: http://jp.physoc.org/content/537/3/1009

Ketone bodies, potential therapeutic uses. - 2001
Veech, R.L. et al., 2001.
IUBMB life, 51(4), pp.241–247.
Available at: http://www.ncbi.nlm.nih.gov/pubmed/11569918

Experience with the ketogenic diet in infants. - 2001
Nordli, D.R. et al., 2001.
Pediatrics, 108(1), pp.129–133.
Available at: http://www.ncbi.nlm.nih.gov/pubmed/11433065

Postprandial de novo lipogenesis and metabolic changes induced by a high-carbohydrate, low-fat meal in lean and overweight men. - 2001
Marques-Lopes, I. et al., 2001.
The American journal of clinical nutrition, 73(2), pp.253–261.
Available at: http://www.ncbi.nlm.nih.gov/pubmed/11157321

Insulin resistance, dietary cholesterol, and cholesterol concentration in postmenopausal women. - 2001
Reaven, G.M. et al., 2001.
Metabolism: Clinical and Experimental, 50(5), pp.594–597.

Available at: http://www.ncbi.nlm.nih.gov/pubmed/11319723

High-fat diet versus habitual diet prior to carbohydrate loading: effects of exercise metabolism and cycling performance. - 2001
Lambert, E.V. et al., 2001.
International journal of sport nutrition and exercise metabolism, 11(2), pp.209–225.
Available at: http://www.ncbi.nlm.nih.gov/pubmed/11402254

Effects of a high-fat diet on postabsorptive and postprandial testosterone responses to a fat-rich meal. - 2001
Volek, J.S. et al., 2001.
Metabolism: Clinical and Experimental, 50(11), pp.1351–1355.
Available at: http://www.ncbi.nlm.nih.gov/pubmed/11699056

Is a fast necessary when initiating the ketogenic diet? - 2002
Wirrell, E.C. et al., 2002.
Journal of child neurology, 17(3), pp.179–182.
Available at: http://www.ncbi.nlm.nih.gov/pubmed/12026232

A Ketogenic Diet Favorably Affects Serum Biomarkers for Cardiovascular Disease in Normal-Weight Men. - 2002
Sharman, M.J. et al., 2002.
The Journal of Nutrition, 132(7), pp.1879–1885.
Available at: http://jn.nutrition.org/content/132/7/1879

Effects of high-fat and high-carbohydrate diets on metabolism and performance in cycling. - 2002
Rowlands, D.S. & Hopkins, W.G., 2002.
Metabolism: clinical and experimental, 51(6), pp.678–690.
Available at: http://www.ncbi.nlm.nih.gov/pubmed/12037719

Body composition and hormonal responses to a carbohydrate-restricted diet. - 2002
Volek, J.S. et al., 2002.
Metabolism: clinical and experimental, 51(7), pp.864–870.
Available at: http://www.ncbi.nlm.nih.gov/pubmed/12077732

Effect of 6-month adherence to a very low carbohydrate diet program. - 2002
Westman, E.C. et al., 2002.
The American journal of medicine, 113(1), pp.30–36.
Available at: http://www.ncbi.nlm.nih.gov/pubmed/12106620

The effect of carbohydrate and fat variation in euenergetic diets on postabsorptive free fatty acid release. - 2002

Bisschop, P.H. et al., 2002.
The British Journal of Nutrition, 87(6), pp.555–559.
Available at: http://www.ncbi.nlm.nih.gov/pubmed/12067425

Breath acetone is a reliable indicator of ketosis in adults consuming ketogenic meals. - 2002
Musa-Veloso, K., Likhodii, S.S. & Cunnane, S.C., 2002.
The American Journal of Clinical Nutrition, 76(1), pp.65–70.
Available at: http://ajcn.nutrition.org/content/76/1/65

Protein consumption and bone mineral density in the elderly : the Rancho Bernardo Study. - 2002
Promislow, J.H.E. et al., 2002.
American Journal of Epidemiology, 155(7), pp.636–644.
Available at: http://www.ncbi.nlm.nih.gov/pubmed/11914191

Effects of a hypocaloric, low-carbohydrate diet on weight loss, blood lipids, blood pressure, glucose tolerance, and body composition in free-living overweight women. - 2002
Meckling, K.A. et al., 2002.
Canadian journal of physiology and pharmacology, 80(11), pp.1095–1105.
Available at: http://www.ncbi.nlm.nih.gov/pubmed/12489929

Dietary fat is not a major determinant of body fat. - 2002
Willett, W.C. & Leibel, R.L., 2002.
The American Journal of Medicine, 113 Suppl 9B, p.47S–59S.
Available at: http://www.ncbi.nlm.nih.gov/pubmed/12566139

An Isoenergetic Very Low Carbohydrate Diet Improves Serum HDL Cholesterol and triglyceride Concentrations, the Total Cholesterol to HDL Cholesterol Ratio and Postprandial Lipemic Responses Compared with a Low Fat Diet in Normal Weight, Normolipidemic Women. - 2003
Volek, J.S. et al., 2003.
The Journal of Nutrition, 133(9), pp.2756–2761.
Available at: http://jn.nutrition.org/content/133/9/2756

Effects of dietary carbohydrate on the development of obesity in heterozygous Zucker rats. - 2003
Morris, K.L., Namey, T.C. & Zemel, M.B., 2003.
The Journal of Nutritional Biochemistry, 14(1), pp.32–39.
Available at: http://www.ncbi.nlm.nih.gov/pubmed/12559475

Effects of protein vs. carbohydrate-rich diets on fuel utilisation in obese women during weight loss. - 2003
Labayen, I. et al., 2003.
Forum of nutrition, 56, pp.168–170.

Available at: http://www.ncbi.nlm.nih.gov/pubmed/15806847

Application of a ketogenic diet in children with autistic behavior: pilot study. - 2003
Evangeliou, A. et al., 2003.
Journal of Child Neurology, 18(2), pp.113–118.
Available at: http://www.ncbi.nlm.nih.gov/pubmed/12693778

Effect of low-carbohydrate, unlimited calorie diet on the treatment of childhood obesity: a prospective controlled study. - 2003
Bailes, J.R. et al., 2003.
Metabolic Syndrome and Related Disorders, 1(3), pp.221–225.
Available at: http://www.ncbi.nlm.nih.gov/pubmed/18370665

A reduced ratio of dietary carbohydrate to protein improves body composition and blood lipid profiles during weight loss in adult women. - 2003
Layman, D.K. et al., 2003.
The Journal of Nutrition, 133(2), pp.411–417.
Available at: http://www.ncbi.nlm.nih.gov/pubmed/12566476

A Low-Carbohydrate as Compared with a Low-Fat Diet in Severe Obesity. - 2003
Samaha, F.F. et al., 2003.
New England Journal of Medicine, 348(21), pp.2074–2081.
Available at: http://www.nejm.org/doi/full/10.1056/NEJMoa022637

A Randomized Trial Comparing a Very Low Carbohydrate Diet and a Calorie-Restricted Low Fat Diet on Body Weight and Cardiovascular Risk Factors in Healthy Women. - 2003
Brehm, B.J. et al., 2003.
The Journal of Clinical Endocrinology & Metabolism, 88(4), pp.1617–1623.
Available at: http://press.endocrine.org/doi/full/10.1210/jc.2002-021480

Effect of a high-protein, energy-restricted diet on body composition, glycemic control, and lipid concentrations in overweight and obese hyperinsulinemic men and women. - 2003
Farnsworth, E. et al., 2003.
The American Journal of Clinical Nutrition, 78(1), pp.31–39.
Available at: http://www.ncbi.nlm.nih.gov/pubmed/12816768

D-β-Hydroxybutyrate rescues mitochondrial respiration and mitigates features of Parkinson disease. - 2003
Tieu, K. et al., 2003.
Journal of Clinical Investigation, 112(6), pp.892–901.
Available at: http://www.jci.org/articles/view/18797

Perspectives on the metabolic management of epilepsy through dietary reduction of glucose and elevation of ketone bodies. - 2003
Greene, A.E., Todorova, M.T. & Seyfried, T.N., 2003.
Journal of Neurochemistry, 86(3), pp.529–537.
Available at: http://onlinelibrary.wiley.com/doi/10.1046/j.1471-4159.2003.01862.x/abstract

Clinical use of a carbohydrate-restricted diet to treat the dyslipidemia of the metabolic syndrome. - 2003
Hickey, J.T. et al., 2003.
Metabolic Syndrome and Related Disorders, 1(3), pp.227–232.
Available at: http://www.ncbi.nlm.nih.gov/pubmed/18370666

Effects of a low-carbohydrate diet on weight loss and cardiovascular risk factor in overweight adolescents. - 2003
Sondike, S.B., Copperman, N. & Jacobson, M.S., 2003.
The Journal of pediatrics, 142(3), pp.253–258.
Available at: http://www.ncbi.nlm.nih.gov/pubmed/12640371

Ketoacids? Good medicine? - 2003
Cahill, G.F., Jr & Veech, R.L., 2003.
Transactions of the American Clinical and Climatological Association, 114, pp.149–161; discussion 162–163.
Available at: http://www.ncbi.nlm.nih.gov/pubmed/12813917

Effects of dietary fat on muscle substrates, metabolism, and performance in athletes. - 2003
Vogt, M. et al., 2003.
Medicine and Science in Sports and Exercise, 35(6), pp.952–960.
Available at: https://www.ncbi.nlm.nih.gov/pubmed/12783043

Role of glucose and ketone bodies in the metabolic control of experimental brain cancer. - 2003
Seyfried, T.N. et al., 2003.
British Journal of Cancer, 89(7), pp.1375–1382.
Available at: http://www.ncbi.nlm.nih.gov/pmc/articles/PMC2394295/

Effect of a high saturated fat and no-starch diet on serum lipid subfractions in patients with documented atherosclerotic cardiovascular disease. - 2003
Hays, J.H. et al., 2003.
Mayo Clinic Proceedings, 78(11), pp.1331–1336.
Available at: http://www.ncbi.nlm.nih.gov/pubmed/14601690

Efficacy of the Atkins diet as therapy for intractable epilepsy. - 2003

Kossoff, E.H. et al., 2003.
Neurology, 61(12), pp.1789–1791.
Available at: http://www.ncbi.nlm.nih.gov/pubmed/14694049

Long-term effects of a ketogenic diet in obese patients. - 2004
Dashti, H.M. et al., 2004.
Experimental & Clinical Cardiology, 9(3), pp.200–205.
Available at: http://www.ncbi.nlm.nih.gov/pmc/articles/PMC2716748/

Metabolic Effects of the Very-Low-Carbohydrate Diets:
Misunderstood "Villains" of Human Metabolism. - 2004
Manninen, A.H., 2004.
J Int Soc Sports Nutr.
Available at: http://www.ncbi.nlm.nih.gov/pmc/articles/PMC2129159/

The therapeutic implications of ketone bodies: the effects of
ketone bodies in pathological conditions: ketosis, ketogenic diet,
redox states, insulin resistance, and mitochondrial metabolism -
2004
Veech, R.L., 2004.
Prostaglandins, leukotrienes, and essential fatty acids, 70(3), pp.309–319.
Available at: http://www.ncbi.nlm.nih.gov/pubmed/14769489

Very Low-Carbohydrate and Low-Fat Diets Affect Fasting Lipids
and Postprandial Lipemia Differently in Overweight Men. - 2004
Sharman, M.J. et al., 2004.
The Journal of Nutrition, 134(4), pp.880–885.
Available at: http://jn.nutrition.org/content/134/4/880

The diet-heart hypothesis: a critique. - 2004
Weinberg, S.L., 2004.
Journal of the American College of Cardiology, 43(5), pp.731–733.
Available at: http://www.ncbi.nlm.nih.gov/pubmed/14998608

A Low-Carbohydrate, Ketogenic Diet versus a Low-Fat Diet To
Treat Obesity and Hyperlipidemia. A Randomized, Controlled
Trial. - 2004
Yancy, J., William S. et al., 2004.
Annals of Internal Medicine, 140(10), pp.769–777.
Available   at: http://dx.doi.org/10.7326/0003-4819-140-10-200405180-
00006

Comparison of a very low-carbohydrate and low-fat diet on
fasting lipids, LDL subclasses, insulin resistance, and
postprandial lipemic responses in overweight women. - 2004
Volek, J.S. et al., 2004.
Journal of the American College of Nutrition, 23(2), pp.177–184.

Available at: http://www.ncbi.nlm.nih.gov/pubmed/15047685

The Effects of Low-Carbohydrate versus Conventional Weight Loss Diets in Severely Obese Adults: One-Year Follow-up of a Randomized Trial. - 2004
Stern, L. et al., 2004.
Annals of Internal Medicine, 140(10), pp.778–785.
Available at: http://dx.doi.org/10.7326/0003-4819-140-10-200405180-00007

High intake of cholesterol results in less atherogenic low-density lipoprotein particles in men and women independent of response classification. - 2004
Herron, K.L. et al., 2004.
Metabolism: clinical and experimental, 53(6), pp.823–830.
Available at: http://www.ncbi.nlm.nih.gov/pubmed/15164336

Effects of β-hydroxybutyrate on cognition in memory-impaired adults. - 2004
Reger, M.A. et al., 2004.
Neurobiology of Aging, 25(3), pp.311–314.
Available at:
http://www.sciencedirect.com/science/article/pii/S0197458003000873

Effect of a high-protein, low-carbohydrate diet on blood glucose control in people with type 2 diabetes. - 2004
Gannon, M.C. & Nuttall, F.Q., 2004.
Diabetes, 53(9), pp.2375–2382.
Available at: http://www.ncbi.nlm.nih.gov/pubmed/15331548

Ketogenic diets and physical performance. - 2004
Phinney, S.D., 2004.
Nutrition & Metabolism, 1(1), p.2.
Available at: http://www.nutritionandmetabolism.com/content/1/1/2

The national cholesterol education program diet vs a diet lower in carbohydrates and higher in protein and monounsaturated fat: A randomized trial. - 2004
Aude Y et al., 2004.
Archives of Internal Medicine, 164(19), pp.2141–2146.
Available at:http://dx.doi.org/10.1001/archinte.164.19.2141

Effects of dietary glycaemic index on adiposity, glucose homoeostasis, and plasma lipids in animals. - 2004
Pawlak, D.B., Kushner, J.A. & Ludwig, D.S., 2004.
Lancet, 364(9436), pp.778–785.
Available at: http://www.ncbi.nlm.nih.gov/pubmed/15337404

Dietary fats, carbohydrate, and progression of coronary atherosclerosis in postmenopausal women. - 2004
Mozaffarian, D., Rimm, E.B. & Herrington, D.M., 2004.
The American Journal of Clinical Nutrition, 80(5), pp.1175–1184.
Available at: http://ajcn.nutrition.org/content/80/5/1175

High-Protein, Low-Fat Diets Are Effective for Weight Loss and Favorably Alter Biomarkers in Healthy Adults. - 2004
Johnston, C.S., Tjonn, S.L. & Swan, P.D., 2004.
The Journal of Nutrition, 134(3), pp.586–591.
Available at: http://jn.nutrition.org/content/134/3/586

Comparison of energy-restricted very low-carbohydrate and low-fat diets on weight loss and body composition in overweight men and women. - 2004
Volek, J. et al., 2004.
Nutrition & Metabolism, 1, p.13.
Available at: http://www.ncbi.nlm.nih.gov/pmc/articles/PMC538279/

The antidepressant properties of the ketogenic diet. - 2004
Murphy, P. et al., 2004.
Biological psychiatry, 56(12), pp.981–983.'
Available at: http://www.ncbi.nlm.nih.gov/pubmed/15601609

Is a Calorie Really a Calorie? Metabolic Advantage of Low-Carbohydrate Diets. - 2004
Manninen, A.H., 2004.
Journal of the International Society of Sports Nutrition, 1(2), p.21.
Available at: http://www.jissn.com/content/1/2/21/abstract

Dietary carbohydrates and glycaemic load and the incidence of symptomatic gall stone disease in men. - 2005
Tsai, C.-J. et al., 2005.
Gut, 54(6), pp.823–828.
Available at: http://gut.bmj.com/content/54/6/823

Anti-Angiogenic and Pro-Apoptotic Effects of Dietary Restriction in Experimental Brain Cancer: Role of Glucose and Ketone Bodies. - 2005
Seyfried, T.N. & Mukherjee, P., 2005.
In G. G. Meadows, ed. Integration/Interaction of Oncologic Growth. Cancer Growth and Progression. Springer Netherlands, pp. 259–270.
Available at: http://link.springer.com/chapter/10.1007/1-4020-3414-8_15

Comparison of high-fat and high-protein diets with a high-carbohydrate diet in insulin-resistant obese women. - 2005
McAuley, K.A. et al., 2005.

Diabetologia, 48(1), pp.8–16.
Available at: http://www.ncbi.nlm.nih.gov/pubmed/15616799

Dietary protein and exercise have additive effects on body composition during weight loss in adult women. - 2005
Layman, D.K. et al., 2005.
The Journal of Nutrition, 135(8), pp.1903–1910.
Available at: http://www.ncbi.nlm.nih.gov/pubmed/16046715

Modification of Lipoproteins by Very Low-Carbohydrate Diets. - 2005
Volek, J.S., Sharman, M.J. & Forsythe, C.E., 2005.
The Journal of Nutrition, 135(6), pp.1339–1342.
Available at: http://jn.nutrition.org/content/135/6/1339

The effects of a low-carbohydrate, ketogenic diet on the polycystic ovary syndrome: a pilot study. - 2005
Mavropoulos, J.C. et al., 2005.
Nutrition & metabolism, 2, p.35.
Available at: http://www.ncbi.nlm.nih.gov/pubmed/16359551

Modification of Lipoproteins by Very Low-Carbohydrate Diets. - 2005
Volek, J.S., Sharman, M.J. & Forsythe, C.E., 2005.
The Journal of Nutrition, 135(6), pp.1339–1342.
Available at: http://jn.nutrition.org/content/135/6/1339

Effects of Dietary Carbohydrate Restriction with High Protein Intake on Protein Metabolism and the Somatotropic Axis. - 2005
Harber, M.P. et al., 2005.
The Journal of Clinical Endocrinology & Metabolism, 90(9), pp.5175–5181.
Available at: http://press.endocrine.org/doi/abs/10.1210/jc.2005-0559

Dietary protein intake and renal function. - 2005
Martin, W.F., Armstrong, L.E. & Rodriguez, N.R., 2005.
Nutrition & Metabolism, 2(1), p.25.
Available   at:
http://www.nutritionandmetabolism.com/content/2/1/25/abstract

Macronutrients, fatty acids, cholesterol and prostate cancer risk. - 2005
Bidoli, E. et al., 2005.
Annals of oncology: official journal of the European Society for Medical Oncology / ESMO, 16(1), pp.152–157.
Available at: http://www.ncbi.nlm.nih.gov/pubmed/15598953

Effect of a low-carbohydrate diet on appetite, blood glucose levels, and insulin resistance in obese patients with type 2 diabetes. - 2005
Boden, G. et al., 2005.
Annals of internal medicine, 142(6), pp.403–411.
Available at: http://www.ncbi.nlm.nih.gov/pubmed/15767618

Urinary ketones reflect serum ketone concentration but do not relate to weight loss in overweight premenopausal women following a low-carbohydrate/high-protein diet. - 2005
Coleman, M.D. & Nickols-Richardson, S.M., 2005.
Journal of the American Dietetic Association, 105(4), pp.608–611.
Available at: http://www.ncbi.nlm.nih.gov/pubmed/1580056

Perceived Hunger Is Lower and Weight Loss Is Greater in Overweight Premenopausal Women Consuming a Low-Carbohydrate/High-Protein vs High-Carbohydrate/Low-Fat Diet. - 2005
Nickols-Richardson, S.M. et al., 2005.
Journal of the American Dietetic Association, 105(9), pp.1433–1437.
Available at:http://www.sciencedirect.com/science/article/pii/S000282230501151X

Carbohydrate restriction improves the features of Metabolic Syndrome. Metabolic Syndrome may be defined by the response to carbohydrate restriction. - 2005
Volek, J.S. & Feinman, R.D., 2005.
Nutrition & Metabolism, 2(1), p.31.
Available   at:
http://www.nutritionandmetabolism.com/content/2/1/31/abstract

A low-carbohydrate, ketogenic diet to treat type 2 diabetes. - 2005
Yancy, W.S. et al., 2005.
Nutrition & Metabolism, 2(1), p.34.
Available   at:
http://www.nutritionandmetabolism.com/content/2/1/34/abstract

Short-term effect of eggs on satiety in overweight and obese subjects. - 2005
Vander Wal, J.S. et al., 2005.
Journal of the American College of Nutrition, 24(6), pp.510–515.
Available at: http://www.ncbi.nlm.nih.gov/pubmed/16373948

Separate effects of reduced carbohydrate intake and weight loss on atherogenic dyslipidemia. - 2006
Krauss, R.M. et al., 2006.
The American Journal of Clinical Nutrition, 83(5), pp.1025–1031.

Available at: http://ajcn.nutrition.org/content/83/5/1025

Low carbohydrate diets improve atherogenic dyslipidemia even in the absence of weight loss. - 2006
Feinman, R.D. & Volek, J.S., 2006.
Nutrition & metabolism, 3, p.24.
Available at: http://www.ncbi.nlm.nih.gov/pubmed/16790045

Effects of low-carbohydrate diet and Pycnogenol treatment on retinal antioxidant enzymes in normal and diabetic rats. - 2006
Kamuren, Z.T. et al., 2006.
Journal of Ocular Pharmacology and Therapeutics: The Official Journal of the Association for Ocular Pharmacology and Therapeutics, 22(1), pp.10–18.
Available at: http://www.ncbi.nlm.nih.gov/pubmed/16503770

Dietary treatment of diabetes mellitus in the pre-insulin era (1914-1922) - 2006
Westman, E.C., Yancy, W.S., Jr & Humphreys, M., 2006.
Perspectives in biology and medicine, 49(1), pp.77–83.
Available at: http://www.ncbi.nlm.nih.gov/pubmed/16489278

Dietary cholesterol provided by eggs and plasma lipoproteins in healthy populations. - 2006
Fernandez, M.L., 2006.
Current opinion in clinical nutrition and metabolic care, 9(1), pp.8–12.
Available at: http://www.ncbi.nlm.nih.gov/pubmed/16340654

Effects of low-carbohydrate vs low-fat diets on weight loss and cardiovascular risk factors: A meta-analysis of randomized controlled trials. - 2006
Nordmann AJ et al., 2006.
Archives of Internal Medicine, 166(3), pp.285–293.
Available at: http://dx.doi.org/10.1001/archinte.166.3.285

Short-term effects of severe dietary carbohydrate-restriction advice in Type 2 diabetes—a randomized controlled trial. - 2006
Daly, M.E. et al., 2006.
Diabetic Medicine, 23(1), pp.15–20.
Available at: http://onlinelibrary.wiley.com/doi/10.1111/j.1464-5491.2005.01760.x/abstract

Fuel metabolism in starvation. - 2006
Cahill, G.F., Jr, 2006.
Annual review of nutrition, 26, pp.1–22.
Available at: http://www.ncbi.nlm.nih.gov/pubmed/16848698

Comparison of isocaloric very low carbohydrate/high saturated fat and high carbohydrate/low saturated fat diets on body composition and cardiovascular risk. - 2006
Noakes, M. et al., 2006.
Nutrition & Metabolism, 3(1), p.7.
Available   at:
http://www.nutritionandmetabolism.com/content/3/1/7/abstract

Effects of a carbohydrate-restricted diet on emerging plasma markers for cardiovascular disease. - 2006
Wood, R.J. et al., 2006.
Nutrition & Metabolism, 3(1), p.19.
Available   at:
http://www.nutritionandmetabolism.com/content/3/1/19/abstract

Effects of variation in protein and carbohydrate intake on body mass and composition during energy restriction: a meta-regression. - 2006
Krieger, J.W. et al., 2006.
The American Journal of Clinical Nutrition, 83(2), pp.260–274.
Available at: http://ajcn.nutrition.org/content/83/2/260

A Very Low-Carbohydrate Diet Improves Gastroesophageal Reflux and Its Symptoms. - 2006
Austin, G.L. et al., 2006.
Digestive Diseases and Sciences, 51(8), pp.1307–1312.
Available at: http://link.springer.com/article/10.1007/s10620-005-9027-7

Very-low-carbohydrate diets and preservation of muscle mass. - 2006
Manninen, A.H., 2006.
Nutrition & Metabolism, 3, p.9.
Available at: http://www.ncbi.nlm.nih.gov/pmc/articles/PMC1373635/

A ketogenic diet as a potential novel therapeutic intervention in amyotrophic lateral sclerosis - 2006
Zhao, Z. et al., 2006.
BMC Neuroscience, 7, p.29.
Available at: http://www.ncbi.nlm.nih.gov/pmc/articles/PMC1488864/

Metabolic syndrome is associated with greater histologic severity, higher carbohydrate, and lower fat diet in patients with NAFLD. - 2006
Kang, H. et al., 2006.
The American Journal of Gastroenterology, 101(10), pp.2247–2253.
Available at: http://www.ncbi.nlm.nih.gov/pubmed/17032189

Carbohydrate Restriction Alters Lipoprotein Metabolism by Modifying VLDL, LDL, and HDL Subfraction Distribution and Size in Overweight Men. - 2006
Wood, R.J. et al., 2006.
The Journal of Nutrition, 136(2), pp.384–389.
Available at: http://jn.nutrition.org/content/136/2/384

The effect of a low-carbohydrate diet on bone turnover. - 2006
Carter, J.D., Vasey, F.B. & Valeriano, J., 2006.
Osteoporosis international: a journal established as result of cooperation between the European Foundation for Osteoporosis and the National Osteoporosis Foundation of the USA, 17(9), pp.1398–1403.
Available at: http://www.ncbi.nlm.nih.gov/pubmed/16718399

A low-carbohydrate diet may prevent end-stage renal failure in type 2 diabetes. A case report. - 2006
Nielsen, J.V., Westerlund, P. & Bygren, P., 2006.
Nutrition & Metabolism, 3(1), p.23.
Available   at:
http://www.nutritionandmetabolism.com/content/3/1/23/abstract

Long term effects of ketogenic diet in obese subjects with high cholesterol level. - 2006
Dashti, H.M. et al., 2006.
Molecular and cellular biochemistry, 286(1-2), pp.1–9.
Available at: http://www.ncbi.nlm.nih.gov/pubmed/16652223

Effect of a low-carbohydrate, ketogenic diet program compared to a low-fat diet on fasting lipoprotein subclasses. - 2006
Westman, E.C. et al., 2006.
International journal of cardiology, 110(2), pp.212–216.
Available at: http://www.ncbi.nlm.nih.gov/pubmed/16297472

Effects of low carbohydrate diets high in red meats or poultry, fish and shellfish on plasma lipids and weight loss. - 2007
Cassady, B.A. et al., 2007.
Nutrition & Metabolism, 4, p.23.
Available at: http://www.ncbi.nlm.nih.gov/pubmed/17974023

Essentials of Human Nutrition. - 2007
Jim Mann, A. Stewart Truswell.
Available   at: http://www.amazon.com/Essentials-Human-Nutrition-Jim-Mann/dp/0199290970

Low-carbohydrate nutrition and metabolism. - 2007
Westman, E.C. et al., 2007.
The American Journal of Clinical Nutrition, 86(2), pp.276–284.

Available at: http://ajcn.nutrition.org/content/86/2/276

The Effect of a Low-Carbohydrate, Ketogenic Diet on Nonalcoholic Fatty Liver Disease: A Pilot Study. - 2007
Tendler, D. et al., 2007.
Digestive Diseases and Sciences, 52(2), pp.589–593.
Available at: http://link.springer.com/article/10.1007/s10620-006-9433-5

The Neuropharmacology of the Ketogenic Diet. - 2007
Hartman, A.L. et al., 2007.
Pediatric neurology, 36(5), pp.281–292.
Available at: http://www.ncbi.nlm.nih.gov/pmc/articles/PMC1940242/

The calorically restricted ketogenic diet, an effective alternative therapy for malignant brain cancer. - 2007
Zhou, W. et al., 2007.
Nutrition & Metabolism, 4, p.5.
Available at: http://www.ncbi.nlm.nih.gov/pubmed/17313687

KETONES INHIBIT MITOCHONDRIAL PRODUCTION OF REACTIVE OXYGEN SPECIES PRODUCTION FOLLOWING GLUTAMATE EXCITOTOXICITY BY INCREASING NADH OXIDATION. - 2007
Maalouf, M. et al., 2007.
Neuroscience, 145(1), pp.256–264.
Available at: http://www.ncbi.nlm.nih.gov/pmc/articles/PMC1865572/

Meat, fish and fat intake in relation to subsite-specific risk of colorectal cancer: The Fukuoka Colorectal Cancer Study. - 2007
Kimura, Y. et al., 2007.
Cancer Science, 98(4), pp.590–597.
Available at: http://www.ncbi.nlm.nih.gov/pubmed/17425596

The effects of a low-carbohydrate ketogenic diet and a low-fat diet on mood, hunger, and other self-reported symptoms. - 2007
McClernon, F.J. et al., 2007.
Obesity (Silver Spring, Md.), 15(1), pp.182–187.
Available at: http://www.ncbi.nlm.nih.gov/pubmed/17228046

Beneficial effects of ketogenic diet in obese diabetic subjects. - 2007
Dashti, H.M. et al., 2007.
Molecular and Cellular Biochemistry, 302(1-2), pp.249–256.
Available at: http://www.ncbi.nlm.nih.gov/pubmed/17447017

Comparison of the atkins, zone, ornish, and learn diets for change

in weight and related risk factors among overweight premenopausal women: The a to z weight loss study: a randomized trial. - 2007
Gardner CD et al., 2007.
JAMA, 297(9), pp.969–977.
Available at: http://dx.doi.org/10.1001/jama.297.9.969

A high-fat, ketogenic diet induces a unique metabolic state in mice. - 2007
Kennedy, A.R. et al., 2007.
American Journal of Physiology. Endocrinology and Metabolism, 292(6), pp.E1724–1739.
Available at: http://www.ncbi.nlm.nih.gov/pubmed/17299079

A randomized, crossover comparison of daily carbohydrate limits using the modified Atkins diet. - 2007
Kossoff, E.H. et al., 2007.
Epilepsy & behavior: E&B, 10(3), pp.432–436.
Available at: http://www.ncbi.nlm.nih.gov/pubmed/17324628

Low- and high-carbohydrate weight-loss diets have similar effects on mood but not cognitive performance. - 2007
Halyburton, A.K. et al., 2007.
The American Journal of Clinical Nutrition, 86(3), pp.580–587.
Available at: http://ajcn.nutrition.org/content/86/3/580

Low carbohydrate ketogenic diet enhances cardiac tolerance to global ischaemia. - 2007
Al-Zaid, N.S. et al., 2007.
Acta Cardiologica, 62(4), pp.381–389.
Available at: http://www.ncbi.nlm.nih.gov/pubmed/17824299

Acid-base analysis of individuals following two weight loss diets. - 2007
Yancy, W.S. et al., 2007.
European Journal of Clinical Nutrition, 61(12), pp.1416–1422.
Available at: http://www.ncbi.nlm.nih.gov/pubmed/17299473

A low-carbohydrate diet is more effective in reducing body weight than healthy eating in both diabetic and non-diabetic subjects. - 2007
Dyson, P.A., Beatty, S. & Matthews, D.R., 2007.
Diabetic Medicine, 24(12), pp.1430–1435.
Available at: http://onlinelibrary.wiley.com/doi/10.1111/j.1464-5491.2007.02290.x/abstract

Metabolic Effects of Weight Loss on a Very-Low-Carbohydrate

Diet Compared With an Isocaloric High-Carbohydrate Diet in Abdominally Obese Subjects. - 2008
Tay, J. et al., 2008.
Journal of the American College of Cardiology, 51(1), pp.59–67.
Available at: http://dx.doi.org/10.1016/j.jacc.2007.08.050

Carbohydrate restriction, prostate cancer growth, and the insulin-like growth factor axis. - 2008
Freedland, S.J. et al., 2008.
The Prostate, 68(1), pp.11–19.
Available at: http://www.ncbi.nlm.nih.gov/pubmed/17999389/

Unlimited energy, restricted carbohydrate diet improves lipid parameters in obese children. - 2008
Dunlap, B.S. & Bailes, J.R., 2008.
Metabolic Syndrome and Related Disorders, 6(1), pp.32–36.
Available at: http://www.ncbi.nlm.nih.gov/pubmed/18370834

Effects of a high-protein ketogenic diet on hunger, appetite, and weight loss in obese men feeding ad libitum. - 2008
Johnstone, A.M. et al., 2008.
The American journal of clinical nutrition, 87(1), pp.44–55.
Available at: http://www.ncbi.nlm.nih.gov/pubmed/18175736/

Comparison of low fat and low carbohydrate diets on circulating fatty acid composition and markers of inflammation. - 2008
Forsythe, C.E. et al., 2008.
Lipids, 43(1), pp.65–77.
Available at: http://www.ncbi.nlm.nih.gov/pubmed/18046594

Low-carbohydrate-diet score and risk of type 2 diabetes in women. - 2008
Halton, T.L. et al., 2008.
The American Journal of Clinical Nutrition, 87(2), pp.339–346.
Available at: http://ajcn.nutrition.org/content/87/2/339

Fasting is neuroprotective following traumatic brain injury. - 2008
Davis, L.M. et al., 2008.
Journal of Neuroscience Research, 86(8), pp.1812–1822.
Available at: http://onlinelibrary.wiley.com/doi/10.1002/jnr.21628/abstract

Restricted-carbohydrate diets in patients with type 2 diabetes: a meta-analysis. - 2008
Kirk, J.K. et al., 2008.
Journal of the American Dietetic Association, 108(1), pp.91–100.
Available at: http://www.ncbi.nlm.nih.gov/pubmed/18155993

Antioxidant capacity contributes to protection of ketone bodies against oxidative damage induced during hypoglycemic conditions. - 2008
Haces, M.L. et al., 2008.
Experimental Neurology, 211(1), pp.85–96.
Available at: http://www.ncbi.nlm.nih.gov/pubmed/18339375

Carbohydrate restriction as the default treatment for type 2 diabetes and metabolic syndrome. - 2008
Feinman, R.D. & Volek, J.S., 2008.
Scandinavian cardiovascular journal: SCJ, 42(4), pp.256–263.
Available at: http://www.ncbi.nlm.nih.gov/pubmed/18609058

Ketone bodies as a therapeutic for Alzheimer's disease. - 2008
Henderson, S.T., 2008.
Neurotherapeutics: the journal of the American Society for Experimental NeuroTherapeutics, 5(3), pp.470–480.
Available at: http://www.ncbi.nlm.nih.gov/pubmed/18625458

Effects of weight loss from a very-low-carbohydrate diet on endothelial function and markers of cardiovascular disease risk in subjects with abdominal obesity. - 2008
Keogh, J.B. et al., 2008.
The American Journal of Clinical Nutrition, 87(3), pp.567–576.
Available at: http://ajcn.nutrition.org/content/87/3/567

The ketogenic diet increases mitochondrial glutathione levels - 2008
Jarrett, S.G. et al., 2008.
Journal of neurochemistry, 106(3), pp.1044–1051.
Available at: http://www.ncbi.nlm.nih.gov/pubmed/18466343

Dietary carbohydrate restriction induces a unique metabolic state positively affecting atherogenic dyslipidemia, fatty acid partitioning, and metabolic syndrome. - 2008
Volek, J.S. et al., 2008.
Progress in lipid research, 47(5), pp.307–318.
Available at: http://www.ncbi.nlm.nih.gov/pubmed/18396172

Moderate carbohydrate, moderate protein weight loss diet reduces cardiovascular disease risk compared to high carbohydrate, low protein diet in obese adults: A randomized clinical trial. - 2008
Lasker, D.A.W., Evans, E.M. & Layman, D.K., 2008.
Nutrition & Metabolism, 5, p.30.
Available at: http://www.ncbi.nlm.nih.gov/pubmed/18990242

Effect of the LoBAG30 diet on blood glucose control in people with type 2 diabetes. - 2008
Nuttall, F.Q. et al., 2008.
The British Journal of Nutrition, 99(3), pp.511–519.
Available at: http://www.ncbi.nlm.nih.gov/pubmed/17868489

Ketogenic ratio, calories, and fluids: do they matter? - 2008
Wirrell, E.C., 2008.
Epilepsia, 49 Suppl 8, pp.17–19.
Available at: http://www.ncbi.nlm.nih.gov/pubmed/19049578

Eggs modulate the inflammatory response to carbohydrate restricted diets in overweight men. - 2008
Ratliff, J.C. et al., 2008.
Nutrition & Metabolism, 5, p.6.
Available at: http://www.ncbi.nlm.nih.gov/pubmed/18289377

Spanish Ketogenic Mediterranean diet: a healthy cardiovascular diet for weight loss. - 2008
Pérez-Guisado, J., Muñoz-Serrano, A. & Alonso-Moraga, Á., 2008.
Nutrition Journal, 7(1), p.30.
Available at: http://www.nutritionj.com/content/7/1/30/abstract

Low-carbohydrate diet in type 2 diabetes: stable improvement of bodyweight and glycemic control during 44 months follow-up. - 2008
Nielsen, J.V. & Joensson, E.A., 2008.
Nutrition & Metabolism, 5(1), p.14.
Available   at:
http://www.nutritionandmetabolism.com/content/5/1/14/abstract

Ketogenic diets: additional benefits to the weight loss and unfounded secondary effects - 2008
Pérez-Guisado, J., 2008.
Archivos latinoamericanos de nutrición, 58(4), pp.323–329.
Available at: http://www.ncbi.nlm.nih.gov/pubmed/19368291

The Modified Atkins Diet. - 2008
Kossoff, E.H. & Dorward, J.L., 2008.
Epilepsia, 49, pp.37–41.
Available   at: http://onlinelibrary.wiley.com/doi/10.1111/j.1528-
1167.2008.01831.x/abstract

An isoenergetic high-protein, moderate-fat diet does not compromise strength and fatigue during resistance exercise in women. - 2008
Dipla, K. et al., 2008.

The British Journal of Nutrition, 100(2), pp.283–286.
Available at: https://www.ncbi.nlm.nih.gov/pubmed/18618943

Has carbohydrate-restriction been forgotten as a treatment for diabetes mellitus? A perspective on the ACCORD study design. - 2008
Westman, E.C. & Vernon, M.C., 2008.
Nutrition & Metabolism, 5(1), p.10.
Available   at:
http://www.nutritionandmetabolism.com/content/5/1/10/abstract

Protein-induced satiety: effects and mechanisms of different proteins. - 2008
Veldhorst, M. et al., 2008.
Physiology & behavior, 94(2), pp.300–307.
Available at: http://www.ncbi.nlm.nih.gov/pubmed/18282589/

Targeting energy metabolism in brain cancer with calorically restricted ketogenic diets. - 2008
Seyfried, T.N. et al., 2008.
Epilepsia, 49 Suppl 8, pp.114–116.
Available at: http://www.ncbi.nlm.nih.gov/pubmed/19049606

Hypometabolism as a therapeutic target in Alzheimer's disease. - 2008
Costantini, L.C. et al., 2008.
BMC Neuroscience, 9(Suppl 2), p.S16.
Available at: http://www.biomedcentral.com/1471-2202/9/S2/S16/abstract

The effect of a low-carbohydrate, ketogenic diet versus a low-glycemic index diet on glycemic control in type 2 diabetes mellitus. - 2008
Westman, E.C. et al., 2008.
Nutrition & Metabolism, 5, p.36.
Available at: http://www.ncbi.nlm.nih.gov/pmc/articles/PMC2633336/

Long-term consumption of a carbohydrate-restricted diet does not induce deleterious metabolic effects. - 2008
Grieb, P. et al., 2008.
Nutrition Research, 28(12), pp.825–833.
Available   at:http://www.nrjournal.com/article/S0271-5317(08)00213-3/abstract

Clinical Experience of a Diet Designed to Reduce Aging. - 2009
Rosedale, R., Westman, E.C. & Konhilas, J.P., 2009.
The Journal of Applied Research, 9(4), pp.159–165.
Available at: http://www.ncbi.nlm.nih.gov/pubmed/20204146

Effects of two weight-loss diets on health-related quality of life. - 2009

Yancy, W.S., Jr et al., 2009.
Quality of life research: an international journal of quality of life aspects of treatment, care and rehabilitation, 18(3), pp.281–289.
Available at: http://www.ncbi.nlm.nih.gov/pubmed/19212822/

Effects of a Diet Higher in Carbohydrate/Lower in Fat Versus Lower in Carbohydrate/Higher in Monounsaturated Fat on Postmeal Triglyceride Concentrations and Other Cardiovascular Risk Factors in Type 1 Diabetes. - 2009

Strychar, I. et al., 2009.
Diabetes Care, 32(9), pp.1597–1599.
Available at: http://care.diabetesjournals.org/content/32/9/1597

A moderate-protein diet produces sustained weight loss and long-term changes in body composition and blood lipids in obese adults. - 2009

Layman, D.K. et al., 2009.
The Journal of Nutrition, 139(3), pp.514–521.
Available at: http://www.ncbi.nlm.nih.gov/pubmed/19158228

Effects of a low-carbohydrate diet on glycemic control in outpatients with severe type 2 diabetes. - 2009

Haimoto, H. et al., 2009.
Nutrition & metabolism, 6, p.21.
Available at: http://www.ncbi.nlm.nih.gov/pubmed/19419563

Schizophrenia, gluten, and low-carbohydrate, ketogenic diets: a case report and review of the literature. - 2009

Kraft, B.D. & Westman, E.C., 2009.
Nutrition & Metabolism, 6(1), p.10.
Available   at:
http://www.nutritionandmetabolism.com/content/6/1/10/abstract

Acetoacetate reduces growth and ATP concentration in cancer cell lines which over-express uncoupling protein 2. - 2009

Fine, E.J. et al., 2009.
Cancer Cell International, 9, p.14.
Available at: http://www.ncbi.nlm.nih.gov/pubmed/19480693

Effects of two energy-restricted diets differing in the carbohydrate/protein ratio on weight loss and oxidative changes of obese men. - 2009

Abete, I. et al., 2009.
International Journal of Food Sciences and Nutrition, 60 Suppl 3, pp.1–13.
Available at: http://www.ncbi.nlm.nih.gov/pubmed/18654910

Systematic review of randomized controlled trials of low-carbohydrate vs. low-fat/low-calorie diets in the management of obesity and its comorbidities. - 2009
Hession, M. et al., 2009.
Obesity reviews: an official journal of the International Association for the Study of Obesity, 10(1), pp.36–50.
Available at: http://www.ncbi.nlm.nih.gov/pubmed/18700873

A randomized controlled trial on the efficacy of carbohydrate-reduced or fat-reduced diets in patients attending a telemedically guided weight loss program. - 2009
Frisch, S. et al., 2009.
Cardiovascular Diabetology, 8(1), p.36.
Available at: http://www.cardiab.com/content/8/1/36/abstract

Meta-analysis of animal fat or animal protein intake and colorectal cancer. - 2009
Alexander, D.D. et al., 2009.
The American Journal of Clinical Nutrition, 89(5), pp.1402–1409.
Available at: http://ajcn.nutrition.org/content/89/5/1402

THE NEUROPROTECTIVE PROPERTIES OF CALORIE RESTRICTION, THE KETOGENIC DIET, AND KETONE BODIES. - 2009
Maalouf, M.A., Rho, J.M. & Mattson, M.P., 2009.
Brain research reviews, 59(2), pp.293–315.
Available at: http://www.ncbi.nlm.nih.gov/pmc/articles/PMC2649682/

Carbohydrate Restriction, as a First-Line Dietary Intervention, Effectively Reduces Biomarkers of Metabolic Syndrome in Emirati Adults. - 2009
Al-Sarraj, T. et al., 2009.
The Journal of Nutrition, p.jn.109.109603.
Available   at:
http://jn.nutrition.org/content/early/2009/07/08/jn.109.109603

Long-term effects of a very-low-carbohydrate weight loss diet compared with an isocaloric low-fat diet after 12 mo. - 2009
Brinkworth, G.D. et al., 2009.
The American Journal of Clinical Nutrition, 90(1), pp.23–32.
Available at: http://ajcn.nutrition.org/content/90/1/23

Ketogenic diet reduces cytochrome c release and cellular apoptosis following traumatic brain injury in juvenile rats - 2009
Hu, Z.G. et al., 2009.
Annals of clinical and laboratory science, 39(1), pp.76–83.
Available at: http://www.ncbi.nlm.nih.gov/pubmed/19201746

Carbohydrate Restriction has a More Favorable Impact on the Metabolic Syndrome than a Low Fat Diet. - 2009
Volek, J.S. et al., 2009.
Lipids, 44(4), pp.297–309.
Available at: http://link.springer.com/article/10.1007/s11745-008-3274-2

Effects of a low carbohydrate weight loss diet on exercise capacity and tolerance in obese subjects. - 2009
Brinkworth, G.D. et al., 2009.
Obesity (Silver Spring, Md.), 17(10), pp.1916–1923.
Available at: http://www.ncbi.nlm.nih.gov/pubmed/19373224/

A Very Low-Carbohydrate Diet Improves Symptoms and Quality of Life in Diarrhea-Predominant Irritable Bowel Syndrome. - 2009
Austin, G.L. et al., 2009.
Clinical Gastroenterology and Hepatology, 7(6), pp.706–708.e1.
Available at:http://www.cghjournal.org/article/S1542-3565(09)00198-0/abstract

Sex differences in energy homeostatis following a diet relatively high in protein exchanged with carbohydrate, assessed in a respiration chamber in humans. - 2009
Westerterp-Plantenga, M.S. et al., 2009.
Physiology & Behavior, 97(3-4), pp.414–419.
Available at: http://www.ncbi.nlm.nih.gov/pubmed/19318111

A very low carbohydrate ketogenic diet improves glucose tolerance in ob/ob mice independently of weight loss. - 2009
Badman, M.K. et al., 2009.
American journal of physiology. Endocrinology and metabolism, 297(5), pp.E1197–1204.
Available at: http://www.ncbi.nlm.nih.gov/pubmed/19738035

Effects of meals high in carbohydrate, protein, and fat on ghrelin and peptide YY secretion in prepubertal children. - 2009
Lomenick, J.P. et al., 2009.
The Journal of Clinical Endocrinology and Metabolism, 94(11), pp.4463–4471.
Available at: http://www.ncbi.nlm.nih.gov/pubmed/19820013

Therapeutic role of low-carbohydrate ketogenic diet in diabetes. - 2009
Al-Khalifa, A. et al., 2009.
Nutrition (Burbank, Los Angeles County, Calif.), 25(11-12), pp.1177–1185.
Available at: http://www.ncbi.nlm.nih.gov/pubmed/19818281/

Reduced Pain and Inflammation in Juvenile and Adult Rats Fed a Ketogenic Diet. - 2009
Ruskin, D.N., Kawamura, M., Jr & Masino, S.A., 2009.
PLoS ONE, 4(12), p.e8349.
Available at: http://dx.doi.org/10.1371/journal.pone.0008349

Meta-analysis of prospective cohort studies evaluating the association of saturated fat with cardiovascular disease. - 2010
Siri-Tarino, P.W. et al., 2010.
The American journal of clinical nutrition, 91(3), pp.535–546.
Available at: http://www.ncbi.nlm.nih.gov/pubmed/20071648

Dietary Guidelines for Americans - 2010
Food and Nutrition Information Center, Center for Nutrition Policy and Promotion
United States Department of Agriculture
Available at: http://fnic.nal.usda.gov/dietary-guidance/dietary-guidelines

Renal function following long-term weight loss in individuals with abdominal obesity on a very-low-carbohydrate diet vs high-carbohydrate diet. - 2010
Brinkworth, G.D. et al., 2010.
Journal of the American Dietetic Association, 110(4), pp.633–638.
Available at: http://www.ncbi.nlm.nih.gov/pubmed/20338292

Eggs distinctly modulate plasma carotenoid and lipoprotein subclasses in adult men following a carbohydrate-restricted diet. - 2010
Mutungi, G. et al., 2010.
The Journal of nutritional biochemistry, 21(4), pp.261–267.
Available at: http://www.ncbi.nlm.nih.gov/pubmed/19369056

Resistance training in overweight women on a ketogenic diet conserved lean body mass while reducing body fat. - 2010
Jabekk, P.T. et al., 2010.
Nutrition & Metabolism, 7(1), p.17.
Available   at:
http://www.nutritionandmetabolism.com/content/7/1/17/abstract

Diet-induced ketosis improves cognitive performance in aged rats. - 2010
Xu, K. et al., 2010.
Advances in experimental medicine and biology, 662, pp.71–75.
Available at: http://www.ncbi.nlm.nih.gov/pubmed/20204773

Further decrease in glycated hemoglobin following ingestion of a LoBAG30 diet for 10 weeks compared to 5 weeks in people with

untreated type 2 diabetes. - 2010
Gannon, M.C., Hoover, H. & Nuttall, F.Q., 2010.
Nutrition & Metabolism, 7, p.64.
Available at: http://www.ncbi.nlm.nih.gov/pubmed/20670414

Type 1 diabetes and epilepsy: efficacy and safety of the ketogenic diet. - 2010
Dressler, A. et al., 2010.
Epilepsia, 51(6), pp.1086–1089.
Available at: http://www.ncbi.nlm.nih.gov/pubmed/20345934

Meta-analysis of prospective cohort studies evaluating the association of saturated fat with cardiovascular disease. - 2010
Siri-Tarino, P.W. et al., 2010.
The American Journal of Clinical Nutrition, 91(3), pp.535–546.
Available at: http://ajcn.nutrition.org/content/91/3/535

Metabolic management of glioblastoma multiforme using standard therapy together with a restricted ketogenic diet: Case Report. - 2010
Zuccoli, G. et al., 2010.
Nutrition & Metabolism, 7, p.33.
Available at: http://www.ncbi.nlm.nih.gov/pmc/articles/PMC2874558/

Ketogenic diet slows down mitochondrial myopathy progression in mice. - 2010
Ahola-Erkkilä, S. et al., 2010.
Human Molecular Genetics, 19(10), pp.1974–1984.
Available at: http://hmg.oxfordjournals.org/content/19/10/1974

Long-term outcomes of children treated with the ketogenic diet in the past. - 2010
Patel, A. et al., 2010.
Epilepsia, 51(7), pp.1277–1282.
Available   at: http://onlinelibrary.wiley.com/doi/10.1111/j.1528-1167.2009.02488.x/abstract

Dietary intake of saturated fatty acids and mortality from cardiovascular disease in Japanese: the Japan Collaborative Cohort Study for Evaluation of Cancer Risk (JACC) Study. - 2010
Yamagishi, K. et al., 2010.
The American Journal of Clinical Nutrition, 92(4), pp.759–765.
Available at: http://www.ncbi.nlm.nih.gov/pubmed/20685950

Efficacy and Safety of a High Protein, Low Carbohydrate Diet for Weight Loss in Severely Obese Adolescents. - 2010
Krebs, N.F. et al., 2010.

The Journal of pediatrics, 157(2), pp.252–258.
Available at: http://www.ncbi.nlm.nih.gov/pmc/articles/PMC2892194/

Neuroprotective and Anti-inflammatory Activities of Ketogenic Diet on MPTP-induced Neurotoxicity. - 2010
Yang, X. & Cheng, B., 2010.
Journal of Molecular Neuroscience, 42(2), pp.145–153.
Available at: http://link.springer.com/article/10.1007/s12031-010-9336-y

Presence or absence of carbohydrates and the proportion of fat in a high-protein diet affect appetite suppression but not energy expenditure in normal-weight human subjects fed in energy balance. - 2010
Veldhorst, M.A.B. et al., 2010.
The British journal of nutrition, 104(9), pp.1395–1405.
Available at: http://www.ncbi.nlm.nih.gov/pubmed/20565999

Weight and metabolic outcomes after 2 years on a low-carbohydrate versus low-fat diet: a randomized trial. - 2010
Foster, G.D. et al., 2010.
Annals of internal medicine, 153(3), pp.147–157.
Available at: http://www.ncbi.nlm.nih.gov/pubmed/20679559

Egg consumption as part of an energy-restricted high-protein diet improves blood lipid and blood glucose profiles in individuals with type 2 diabetes. - 2011
Pearce, K.L., Clifton, P.M. & Noakes, M., 2011.
The British journal of nutrition, 105(4), pp.584–592.
Available at: http://www.ncbi.nlm.nih.gov/pubmed/21134328

Mild experimental ketosis increases brain uptake of 11C-acetoacetate and 18F-fluorodeoxyglucose: a dual-tracer PET imaging study in rats. - 2011
Pifferi, F. et al., 2011.
Nutritional Neuroscience, 14(2), pp.51–58.
Available at: https://www.ncbi.nlm.nih.gov/pubmed/21605500

Reversal of Diabetic Nephropathy by a Ketogenic Diet. - 2011
Poplawski, M.M. et al., 2011.
PLoS ONE, 6(4), p.e18604.
Available at: http://dx.doi.org/10.1371/journal.pone.0018604

Lecture Notes: Clinical Biochemistry. - 2011
Geoffrey Beckett, Simon W. Walker, Peter Rae, Peter Ashby.

A carbohydrate-restricted diet during resistance training promotes more favorable changes in body composition and markers of health in obese women with and without insulin resistance. - 2011
Kreider, R.B. et al., 2011.
The Physician and Sportsmedicine, 39(2), pp.27–40.
Available at: http://www.ncbi.nlm.nih.gov/pubmed/21673483

The effect of the Spanish Ketogenic Mediterranean Diet on nonalcoholic fatty liver disease: a pilot study - 2011
Perez-Guisado, J. & Muñoz-Serrano, A., 2011.
Journal of medicinal food, 14(7-8), pp.677–680.
Available at: http://www.ncbi.nlm.nih.gov/pubmed/21688989

A pilot study of the Spanish Ketogenic Mediterranean Diet: an effective therapy for the metabolic syndrome. 2011
Pérez-Guisado, J. & Muñoz-Serrano, A., 2011.
Journal of medicinal food, 14(7-8), pp.681–687.
Available at: http://www.ncbi.nlm.nih.gov/pubmed/21612461

Is There a Role for Carbohydrate Restriction in the Treatment and Prevention of Cancer? - 2011
Rainer J Klement, Ulrike Kämmerer, 2011
Medscape
Available at: http://www.medscape.com/viewarticle/757713_1

Metabolic management of brain cancer. - 2011
Seyfried, T.N. et al., 2011.
Biochimica et Biophysica Acta (BBA) - Bioenergetics, 1807(6), pp.577–594.
Available
at:http://www.sciencedirect.com/science/article/pii/S0005272810006857

A ketogenic diet delays weight loss and does not impair working memory or motor function in the R6/2 1J mouse model of Huntington's disease. - 2011
Ruskin, D.N. et al., 2011.
Physiology & Behavior, 103(5), pp.501–507.
Available at: http://www.ncbi.nlm.nih.gov/pubmed/21501628

Change in food cravings, food preferences, and appetite during a low-carbohydrate and low-fat diet. - 2011
Martin, C.K. et al., 2011.
Obesity (Silver Spring, Md.), 19(10), pp.1963–1970.
Available at: http://www.ncbi.nlm.nih.gov/pubmed/21494226

A Low Carbohydrate, High Protein Diet Slows Tumor Growth and Prevents Cancer Initiation. - 2011
Ho, V.W. et al., 2011.
Cancer Research.
Available   at:
http://cancerres.aacrjournals.org/content/early/2011/06/10/0008-5472.CAN-10-3973

Dietary treatment of epilepsy: rebirth of an ancient treatment. - 2011
Jóźwiak, S., Kossoff, E.H. & Kotulska-Jóźwiak, K., 2011.
Neurologia i neurochirurgia polska, 45(4), pp.370–378.
Available at: http://www.ncbi.nlm.nih.gov/pubmed/22101998

Effect of ketogenic mediterranean diet with phytoextracts and low carbohydrates/high-protein meals on weight, cardiovascular risk factors, body composition and diet compliance in Italian council employees. - 2011
Paoli, A., Cenci, L. & Grimaldi, K.A., 2011.
Nutrition Journal, 10(1), p.112.
Available at: http://www.nutritionj.com/content/10/1/112/abstract

Diet composition modifies the toxicity of repeated soman exposure in rats. - 2011
Langston, J.L. & Myers, T.M., 2011.
Neurotoxicology, 32(6), pp.907–915.
Available at: http://www.ncbi.nlm.nih.gov/pubmed/21641933

Low carbohydrate ketogenic diet prevents the induction of diabetes using streptozotocin in rats. - 2011
Al-Khalifa, A. et al., 2011.
Experimental and Toxicologic Pathology, 63(7–8), pp.663–669.
Available   at:
http://www.sciencedirect.com/science/article/pii/S0940299310000862

Adiponectin changes in relation to the macronutrient composition of a weight-loss diet. - 2011
Summer, S.S. et al., 2011.
Obesity (Silver Spring, Md.), 19(11), pp.2198–2204.
Available at: http://www.ncbi.nlm.nih.gov/pubmed/21455123

Metabolic impact of a ketogenic diet compared to a hypocaloric diet in obese children and adolescents. - 2012
Partsalaki, I., Karvela, A. & Spiliotis, B.E., 2012.
Journal of pediatric endocrinology & metabolism: JPEM, 25(7-8), pp.697–704.
Available at: http://www.ncbi.nlm.nih.gov/pubmed/23155696

Comparative effects of low-carbohydrate high-protein versus low-fat diets on the kidney. - 2012
Friedman, A.N. et al., 2012.
Clinical journal of the American Society of Nephrology: CJASN, 7(7), pp.1103–1111.
Available at: http://www.ncbi.nlm.nih.gov/pubmed/22653255

Effects of low-carbohydrate diets versus low-fat diets on metabolic risk factors: a meta-analysis of randomized controlled clinical trials. - 2012
Hu, T. et al., 2012.
American Journal of Epidemiology, 176 Suppl 7, pp.S44–54.
Available at: http://www.ncbi.nlm.nih.gov/pubmed/23035144

Medium term effects of a ketogenic diet and a Mediterranean diet on resting energy expenditure and respiratory ratio. - 2012
Paoli, A. et al., 2012.
BMC Proceedings, 6(Suppl 3), p.P37.
Available at: http://www.biomedcentral.com/1753-6561/6/S3/P37

Marks' Basic Medical Biochemistry. - 2012
Alisa Peet MD et al.
Available   at: http://www.amazon.com/Marks-Medical-Biochemistry-Lieberman-Markss/dp/160831572X

Nutrition and Acne: Therapeutic Potential of Ketogenic Diets. - 2012

Paoli, A. et al., 2012.
Skin Pharmacology and Physiology, 25(3), pp.111–117.
Available at: http://www.karger.com/Article/FullText/336404

Ketogenic diet does not affect strength performance in elite artistic gymnasts. - 2012
Paoli, A. et al., 2012.
Journal of the International Society of Sports Nutrition, 9, p.34.
Available at: http://www.ncbi.nlm.nih.gov/pmc/articles/PMC3411406/

Caprylic triglyceride as a novel therapeutic approach to effectively improve the performance and attenuate the symptoms due to the motor neuron loss in ALS disease. - 2012
Zhao, W. et al., 2012.
PloS One, 7(11), p.e49191.
Available at: http://www.ncbi.nlm.nih.gov/pubmed/23145119

The Ketogenic Diet Is an Effective Adjuvant to Radiation Therapy for the Treatment of Malignant Glioma. - 2012
Abdelwahab, M.G. et al., 2012.
PLoS ONE, 7(5), p.e36197.
Available at: http://dx.doi.org/10.1371/journal.pone.0036197

The ketogenic diet as a treatment paradigm for diverse neurological disorders. - 2012
Stafstrom, C.E. & Rho, J.M., 2012.
Frontiers in Pharmacology, 3, p.59.
Available at: http://www.ncbi.nlm.nih.gov/pubmed/22509165

Targeting insulin inhibition as a metabolic therapy in advanced cancer: a pilot safety and feasibility dietary trial in 10 patients. - 2012
Fine, E.J. et al., 2012.
Nutrition (Burbank, Los Angeles County, Calif.), 28(10), pp.1028–1035.
Available at: http://www.ncbi.nlm.nih.gov/pubmed/22840388

Effects of dietary composition on energy expenditure during weight-loss maintenance. - 2012
Ebbeling, C.B. et al., 2012.
JAMA: the journal of the American Medical Association, 307(24), pp.2627–2634.
Available at: http://www.ncbi.nlm.nih.gov/pubmed/22735432

Effect of low-calorie versus low-carbohydrate ketogenic diet in type 2 diabetes. - 2012
Hussain, T.A. et al., 2012.
Nutrition, 28(10), pp.1016–1021.

Available at: http://www.nutritionjrnl.com/article/S0899-9007(12)00073-1/abstract

Gluconeogenesis and protein-induced satiety. - 2012
Veldhorst, M.A.B., Westerterp, K.R. & Westerterp-Plantenga, M.S., 2012.
British Journal of Nutrition, 107(04), pp.595–600.
Availalbe at: http://journals.cambridge.org/action/displayAbstract?fromPage=online&aid=8483003&fileId=S0007114511003254

The ketogenic diet increases brain glucose and ketone uptake in aged rats: a dual tracer PET and volumetric MRI study. - 2012
Roy, M. et al., 2012.
Brain Research, 1488, pp.14–23.
Available at: https://www.ncbi.nlm.nih.gov/pubmed/23063891

Effects of Dietary Composition During Weight Loss Maintenance: A Controlled Feeding Study. - 2012
Ebbeling, C.B. et al., 2012.
JAMA: the journal of the American Medical Association, 307(24), pp.2627–2634.
Available at: http://www.ncbi.nlm.nih.gov/pmc/articles/PMC3564212/

Suppression of oxidative stress by β-hydroxybutyrate, an endogenous histone deacetylase inhibitor. - 2013
Shimazu, T. et al., 2013.
Science (New York, N.Y.), 339(6116), pp.211–214.
Available at: http://www.ncbi.nlm.nih.gov/pubmed/23223453

Biochemistry - 2013
Denise R. Ferrier PhD
Available at: http://www.amazon.com/Biochemistry-Lippincotts-Illustrated-Reviews-Series/dp/1451175620

Macronutrients and Obesity: Revisiting the Calories in, Calories out Framework - 2013
Riera-Crichton, D. & Tefft, N., 2013.
Rochester, NY: Social Science Research Network.
Available at: http://papers.ssrn.com/abstract=2279503

Therapeutic ketosis with ketone ester delays central nervous system oxygen toxicity seizures in rats. - 2013
D'Agostino, D.P. et al., 2013.
American Journal of Physiology - Regulatory, Integrative and Comparative Physiology, 304(10), pp.R829–R836.
Available at: http://ajpregu.physiology.org/content/304/10/R829

Ketogenic Diets Enhance Oxidative Stress and Radio-Chemo-Therapy Responses in Lung Cancer Xenografts. - 2013
Allen, B.G. et al., 2013.
Clinical Cancer Research, 19(14), pp.3905–3913.
Available at: http://clincancerres.aacrjournals.org/content/19/14/3905

Beyond weight loss: a review of the therapeutic uses of very-low-carbohydrate (ketogenic) diets. - 2013
Paoli, A. et al., 2013.
European Journal of Clinical Nutrition, 67(8), pp.789–796.
Available   at:
http://www.nature.com/ejcn/journal/v67/n8/full/ejcn2013116a.html

The Ketogenic Diet and Hyperbaric Oxygen Therapy Prolong Survival in Mice with Systemic Metastatic Cancer. - 2013
Poff, A.M. et al., 2013.
PLoS ONE, 8(6), p.e65522.
Available at: http://dx.doi.org/10.1371/journal.pone.0065522

The ketogenic diet for type II bipolar disorder. - 2013
Phelps, J.R., Siemers, S.V. & El-Mallakh, R.S., 2013.
Neurocase, 19(5), pp.423–426.
Available at: http://dx.doi.org/10.1080/13554794.2012.690421

Treatment of diabetes and diabetic complications with a ketogenic diet - 2013
Mobbs, C.V. et al., 2013.
Journal of child neurology, 28(8), pp.1009–1014.
Available at: http://www.ncbi.nlm.nih.gov/pubmed/23680948

Effects of a short-term carbohydrate-restricted diet on strength and power performance. - 2013
Sawyer, J.C. et al., 2013.
Journal of Strength and Conditioning Research / National Strength & Conditioning Association, 27(8), pp.2255–2262.
Available at: http://www.ncbi.nlm.nih.gov/pubmed/23774282

Short term improvement of migraine headaches during ketogenic diet: a prospective observational study in a dietician clinical setting. - 2013
Di Lorenzo, C. et al., 2013.
The Journal of Headache and Pain, 14(Suppl 1), p.P219.
Available at: http://www.ncbi.nlm.nih.gov/pmc/articles/PMC3620251/

Ketosis proportionately spares glucose utilization in brain. - 2013
Zhang, Y. et al., 2013.

Journal of Cerebral Blood Flow and Metabolism: Official Journal of the International Society of Cerebral Blood Flow and Metabolism, 33(8), pp.1307–1311.
Available at: https://www.ncbi.nlm.nih.gov/pubmed/23736643

Ketosis and appetite-mediating nutrients and hormones after weight loss. - 2013
Sumithran, P. et al., 2013.
European journal of clinical nutrition, 67(7), pp.759–764.
Available at: http://www.ncbi.nlm.nih.gov/pubmed/23632752/

Ketogenic diets and thermal pain: dissociation of hypoalgesia, elevated ketones, and lowered glucose in rats. - 2013
Ruskin, D.N. et al., 2013.
The Journal of Pain: Official Journal of the American Pain Society, 14(5), pp.467–474.
Available at: http://www.ncbi.nlm.nih.gov/pubmed/23499319

SFAs do not impair endothelial function and arterial stiffness. - 2013
Sanders, T.A. et al., 2013.
The American Journal of Clinical Nutrition, 98(3), pp.677–683.
Available at: http://ajcn.nutrition.org/content/98/3/677

Ketogenic diet improves core symptoms of autism in BTBR mice. - 2013
Ruskin, D.N. et al., 2013.
PloS One, 8(6), p.e65021.
Available at: http://www.ncbi.nlm.nih.gov/pubmed/23755170

Very-low-carbohydrate ketogenic diet v. low-fat diet for long-term weight loss: a meta-analysis of randomised controlled trials. - 2013
Bueno, N.B. et al., 2013.
The British journal of nutrition, 110(7), pp.1178–1187.
Available at: http://www.ncbi.nlm.nih.gov/pubmed/23651522

Ketogenic Diet Improves Forelimb Motor Function after Spinal Cord Injury in Rodents. - 2013
Streijger, F. et al., 2013.
PLoS ONE, 8(11).
Available at: http://www.ncbi.nlm.nih.gov/pmc/articles/PMC3817084/

Assessment of insulin resistance and metabolic syndrome in drug naive patients of bipolar disorder. - 2014
Guha, P. et al., 2014.
Indian journal of clinical biochemistry: IJCB, 29(1), pp.51–56.

Available at: http://www.ncbi.nlm.nih.gov/pubmed/24478549

Ketone supplementation decreases tumor cell viability and prolongs survival of mice with metastatic cancer - 2014
Poff, A.M. et al., 2014.
International journal of cancer. Journal international du cancer.
Available at: http://www.ncbi.nlm.nih.gov/pubmed/24615175

Calories, carbohydrates, and cancer therapy with radiation: exploiting the five R's through dietary manipulation. - 2014
Klement, R.J. & Champ, C.E., 2014.
Cancer Metastasis Reviews.
Available at: http://www.ncbi.nlm.nih.gov/pubmed/24436017

Cancer as a metabolic disease: implications for novel therapeutics. - 2014
Seyfried, T.N. et al., 2014.
Carcinogenesis, 35(3), pp.515–527.
Available at: http://carcin.oxfordjournals.org/content/35/3/515

A non-calorie-restricted low-carbohydrate diet is effective as an alternative therapy for patients with type 2 diabetes. - 2014
Yamada, Y. et al., 2014.
Internal medicine (Tokyo, Japan), 53(1), pp.13–19.
Available at: http://www.ncbi.nlm.nih.gov/pubmed/24390522

Low-carbohydrate/high-protein diet improves diastolic cardiac function and the metabolic syndrome in overweight-obese patients with type 2 diabetes. - 2014
Von Bibra, H. et al., 2014.
IJC Metabolic & Endocrine, 2, pp.11–18.
Available at: http://www.ijcme-journal.com/article/S2214762413000078/abstract

Inhibition of fluorescent advanced glycation end products (AGEs) of human serum albumin upon incubation with 3-β-hydroxybutyrate. - 2014
Bohlooli, M. et al., 2014.
Molecular biology reports, 41(6), pp.3705–3713.
Available at: http://www.ncbi.nlm.nih.gov/pubmed/24535268

A Randomized Pilot Trial of a Moderate Carbohydrate Diet Compared to a Very Low Carbohydrate Diet in Overweight or Obese Individuals with Type 2 Diabetes Mellitus or Prediabetes. - 2014
Saslow, L.R. et al., 2014.
PLoS ONE, 9(4), p.e91027.

Available at: http://dx.doi.org/10.1371/journal.pone.0091027

Risk of Breast Cancer Recurrence Associated with Carbohydrate Intake and Tissue Expression of IGF-1 Receptor. - 2014
Emond, J.A. et al., 2014.
Cancer Epidemiology Biomarkers & Prevention, p.cebp.1218.2013.
Available at: http://cebp.aacrjournals.org/content/early/2014/04/22/1055-9965.EPI-13-1218

Effects of a eucaloric reduced-carbohydrate diet on body composition and fat distribution in women with PCOS. - 2014
Goss, A.M. et al., 2014.
Metabolism - Clinical and Experimental.
Available   at:
http://www.metabolismjournal.com/article/S0026049514002108/abstract

Return of hunger following a relatively high carbohydrate breakfast is associated with earlier recorded glucose peak and nadir. - 2014
Chandler-Laney, P.C. et al., 2014.
Appetite, 80C, pp.236–241.
Available at: http://www.ncbi.nlm.nih.gov/pubmed/24819342

The contribution of ketone bodies to basal and activity-dependent neuronal oxidation in vivo. - 2014
Chowdhury, G.M. et al., 2014.
Journal of Cerebral Blood Flow and Metabolism: Official Journal of the International Society of Cerebral Blood Flow and Metabolism, 34(7), pp.1233–1242.
Available at: http://www.ncbi.nlm.nih.gov/pubmed/24780902

Long-term effects of a ketogenic diet on body composition and bone mineralization in GLUT-1 deficiency syndrome: a case series. - 2014
Bertoli, S. et al., 2014.
Nutrition (Burbank, Los Angeles County, Calif.), 30(6), pp.726–728.
Available at: http://www.ncbi.nlm.nih.gov/pubmed/24800673

Index

acidosis, 41, 53, 146-147, 158

acne, 56, 58

adiponectin, 81, 84, 90, 137, 142, 143

advaced glycation end-products (AGEs), 39, 145

aging, 79, 96, 217

alzheimers, 39, 45, 46, 49, 52, 54, 56, 90, 97, 206, 209, 213, 215, 219

amyotrophic lateral sclerosis (ALS), 56, 100, 239

anti-oxidants, 52, 91, 135, 139, 211, 213

apoliproteins (apoB, etc), 25, 72, 113, 114, 126, 129, 132, 139, 159

appetite, 224-232

atherogenic dyslipidemia, 48, 53, 73, 116, 123, 126, 127, 132, 133, 134, 138, 174, 265

atherosclerosis, 18, 39, 69, 112, 119, 124, 172

ATP, 47, 56, 94, 212, 220, 248

autism, 16, 56, 57, 104, 207, 220, 223

bipolar disorder, 37, 223

blood pH, 11, 131, 196

blood pressure, 26, 27, 31, 32, 39, 42, 53, 67, 71, 75, 77, 80, 81, 85, 116, 135-137, 140-142, 144, 158, 159, 185, 200, 223

brachial artery flow-mediated dilation, 133

cachexia (wasting syndrome), 83, 242

calcium, 5, 87, 212, 233, 234, 237

cataracts, 91

cortisol, 11, 14, 27

creatinine, 24, 29, 33, 36

CRP, 74, 117, 127, 135, 136, 144

cytochrome C release, 95, 97, 216, 217

energy expenditure, 19, 34, 35, 36, 50, 82, 93, 147, 169, 189, 199, 200, 229, 231

fatigue, 23, 51, 77, 242

fatty liver disease, 23, 32, 128, 258-260

free radical formation, 46, 47, 49, 92, 211

gall bladder and stones, 70, 256-258

GGT, 142

glucagon, 6, 27, 43-44, 62-64, 68-69, 136, 151, 224, 261-262

glucose trasporter 1 (GLUT-1) deficiency syndrome, 60, 241

glutathione, 52, 211

glycogen, 7, 10, 13, 18, 88-89, 193-195, 197-199

glycolysis, 57, 59, 69, 102, 220, 243-244, 247-249, 253

glycosuria, 147, 152

hemoglobin A1c (HbA1c), 21, 24, 36, 40, 66, 68, 71, 76-77, 85, 87, 122, 144, 150-158, 192

homeostatis model analysis-insulin resistance (HOMA-IR), 120, 128, 143, 223, 258

homocysteine, 27, 136

Huntington's Disease, 98-99, 219

hypercapnia (elevated blood CO_2), 9, 65

hypercholesterolemia, 49, 110-111, 120

hypertension, 75

injury recovery, 55, 57, 95, 104-105, 212, 216, 241

insulin, 6, 10-11, 14-15, 19-20, 27, 35, 42-43, 49, 53, 56, 62-69, 76, 78-79, 81, 83, 90, 94, 100, 113, 120, 122, 128, 134, 136-139, 143-144, 147-152, 154-156, 159, 196, 203, 212, 223-225, 228, 232, 247-248, 251, 254, 261-263, 265

insulin resistance, 19-20, 27, 49, 56, 72, 85, 115, 122, 132, 145, 175, 223

insulin sensitivity, 19, 71, 83, 115, 122, 138, 143, 151, 248, 264-265

insulin-like growth factor 1 (IGF-1), 56, 83, 86, 94, 247-248, 254

insulin:glucagon ratio, 6, 43, 62-63, 69, 151, 261

Summary

There's no such thing as an essential carbohydrate.

~ The End ~

CPSIA information can be obtained at www.ICGtesting.com
Printed in the USA
LVOW04s1029240415

435961LV00016B/168/P